SENSIBLE LIVING

SENSIBLE LIVING

Winning Your Fight Against Arthritis

VIRGIL HARBERT

WILLIAM MORROW
AND COMPANY, INC.
New York

Library of Congress Cataloging-in-Publication Data

Harbert, Virgil.
Sensible living : winning your fight against arthritis / Virgil
Harbert.
p.   cm.
ISBN 0-688-07821-4
1. Harbert, Virgil—Health. 2. Arthritis—Patients—United
States—Biography. 3. Arthritis—Exercise therapy. I. Title.
RC933.H34 1988
616.7'22'00924—dc 19
[B]   88-19091
CIP

Printed in the United States of America

First Edition

1 2 3 4 5 6 7 8 9 10

BOOK DESIGN BY RICHARD ORIOLO

I would like to dedicate this book to Anna Uhrich, the retired nurse who got me started exercising, and to Anne Anderson, account executive for G. F. Thomsen & Associates. She has worked so hard to get this book published. Oftentimes, when I became discouraged, she would call me and give me some good news. If it hadn't been for Anne, I might have given up long ago.

Preface

I want! Everyone wants. Beats there a heart so dead that never to itself hath said, "I have no desires. I have no wants. I need nothing from life."

My benefactors, G. F. Thomsen and Associates, of Mitchell, South Dakota, have taken on the task of finding a writer who can paint a word picture of my life.

I want my true story told, in such a way as to inspire a few of the other thirty million arthritics in the United States to fight this dread disease, through what I call *Sensible Living*. I want to pass on to others that which was given to me by others, the manifold benefits of regular exercise.

In recent years, many scientific studies have been made, by people far smarter than I, concerning the kind and extent of exercise that people should undertake.

I am not a professional. I am not a doctor. I have no degrees in physical therapy. But I discovered what regular, slow-moving exercise could do for me, after I had fought a losing battle for thirty-two years and had sunk to the bottom of the pit of self-pity and self-recrimination. From the bottom of a pit, all you can see is light, but you have to look up. Then and only then could I see my way out.

Thanks to my new-found friends in the Retired Senior Volunteer Program (RSVP), I found I was no longer alone in this battle. Regular exercise was working for me. I began to read every article I could find concerning exercise. I became a walking, talking, breathing, preaching advocate of the type of exercise that senior citizens and beginners can do, without breaking bones that have been weakened by osteoperosis, without straining muscles that have never been exercised before, without bringing further injury to bad backs, and without putting too much strain on the heart.

With the aid of my friends, in our exercise class, I have regained my mobility and my self-esteem. After each exercise session, I have a feeling of exhilaration, and all members of my class tell me the same.

The key word here is regularity. If you wish to follow my lead, you must make regular exercise your first priority. Other activities must come second. We must overcome our inherent laziness.

God put me on His good green earth. It is my wish to live a high-quality life here, as long as He permits.

I want!

VIRGIL HARBERT
May 5, 1988
Mitchell, SD

Contents

1   *Forty-two Years of Struggle:*
    The Beginning, 1945   13

2   *Hard Work and Hard Times: 1946–1949*   21

3   *The Biggest Gamble on the Face of the Earth*   27

4   *Mink Mama, Sand Man, Salesman, Trucker*   33

5   *1958: Looking at Partial Disability*
    and War Wounds   37

6   *My Last Two Jobs: Early Retirement*   43

7   *My Total Disability: When You Hit Bottom,*
    the Only Way to Go Is Up   47

8   *I Do-si-do My Way to Exercise Class*   53

9   *Stress, Relaxation, and Letting Go*   57

10 *Stretching and Flexing Lead to a*
    New Chapter in My Life   63

11 *My Sense of Humor Gets a Workout*   71

12 *Mitchell's Exercise Guru*   79

13 *One Thing Leads to Another: My Video
    and Weight Control*   85

14 *Fresh Out of Excuses: How Other People
    Have Used My Program*   91

15 *Be Patient: God Isn't Through with Me Yet:
    My Life Today*   97

    Exercise Section   105

SENSIBLE LIVING

1

Forty-two Years of Struggle: The Beginning, 1945

I've been fighting arthritis for over forty-two years. During the first thirty-two years of my disease, I was fighting a losing battle. My arthritis got steadily worse. But in the past ten-plus years, I've been winning the battle through sensible living and sensible exercise.

In all my years of struggle, I never gave up hope for recovery. People around here say that the Harberts have a stubborn streak a mile wide. That's true. Stubbornness gave me the courage to look for hope, even when everyone else thought my situation was hopeless.

In 1977, when I was sixty years old, I hit bottom. My arthritis was out of control. My condition had deteriorated to the point that I could no longer feed myself. I had to lean over the table, halfway to my plate, because my arms were too stiff to lift a spoon to my mouth. I could no longer walk, I shuffled. I stooped over. When I

13

was a young man, I was five feet six. In 1977, the joints in my back and knees had been squeezed together so that I was much shorter—five feet three and a half inches. As you might imagine, I was in constant pain. Social Security gave me total disability status. But I still had hope that I would find a way to reverse and reduce the terrible effects of my arthritis.

This is the story of how that happened, the story of my recovery. Most of all it is the story of hope. That's what makes me tick. Hope.

My main aim and thought is to help those who need help most. Most of the people in my exercise class are suffering from one ailment or another. I keep our routine at a pace that anyone can follow. Everyone needs exercise. You know, sometimes I see famous people on TV and when I hear them say they've paid their dues, I think about all the people I know who've paid their dues but aren't famous. Some of these people are barely getting by. Some disabled, some of them are suffering from arthritis. These are the people I want to help. I know them and love them because I am one of them.

So this is my story. I hope it will give hope to people who have almost given up—who are afraid there's no hope left. Somebody told me, "Courage is fear that's said its prayers." Courage, stubbornness, and hope!

My First Attack Hits Me Hard

My arthritis first hit me right after I got out of the the service, after World War II. I've heard it said that arthritis strikes us first at the place of a previous injury. This may not be true for everyone but it was for me. My arthritis started in my knees and when I was in the service, I had sustained a knee injury in parachute school. I was also wounded in the Battle of the Bulge.

So I'll skip over my childhood on the farm in South Dakota and, for now, my experiences in World War II, and start my story with my return home after the war.

My Discharge from the United States Army Paratroopers

On September 25, 1945, I was discharged from the United States Army Paratroopers at Camp McCoy, Wisconsin. I was given a physical exam before being discharged. The doctors were concerned because I had a bad limp from the wound I got from a mortar shell at the Battle of the Bulge. I dragged my left leg slightly. The doctors asked me if I wanted to make a claim for disability. I said no. I was scared they would put me in a hospital and try to cure me of my limp. I didn't want to spend time in a hospital. I wanted to go home. In fact, I was in a hurry to get home. I was happy just to be alive. I was happy my dog tags weren't being sent to my parents, along with my body in a coffin.

I didn't even think to ask them about the long-term effects of my knee injury. I was "Nervous in the Service" and I wanted out!

Mitchell, South Dakota, Home of the Corn Palace

I arrived home in Mitchell during Corn Palace Week. This is our biggest week of the year, a harvest festival in the fall. The Corn Palace—a huge auditorium with towers and turrets—is decorated with corn and grain each year at this time to celebrate the earth's bounty. The festival is our main tourist attraction, and I've always enjoyed it.

That year, 1945, my brother-in-law was a carnie. He owned a string game. "Pull the string and win a prize every time." Of course, some of the prizes were very small. I found his booth at the carnival, threw my barracks bag in his joint, and hurried to use a phone. I called my cousin who lived in Alexandria, seventeen miles east of Mitchell. He dropped everything and gave me a ride home.

We celebrated that night, and the next day I was ready to help my father with the farm work. I had been in partnership with my father before I was drafted and I had continued to send him money while I was in the service. We were poor people and I knew the value of a dollar. I didn't throw much away going out on passes with the other soldiers.

We had an eight-hundred-acre farm. Nowadays, that would be considered small because the size of farms has increased. But at that time we were one of the big farmers. My father and I had a good arrangement. He ran around doing the business and I did most of the work. I enjoyed hard work.

My first chore when I got up the next morning was to relieve my father on the tractor. He was doing some fall plowing. It felt so good to be on that tractor. I thanked God to be home and alive. The hot afternoon sun warmed me all over. The soft, fall breeze flowed gently against my face. The smell of the black loam soil being turned over by the plow was the sweetest smell in the world, I thought. War stinks. I never wanted to see it again.

With the Corn, Comes the First Blizzard and My First Attack

Soon it was time to harvest our corn. That presented something of a problem. We didn't have a mechanical corn picker. There had been a shortage of farm machinery, be-

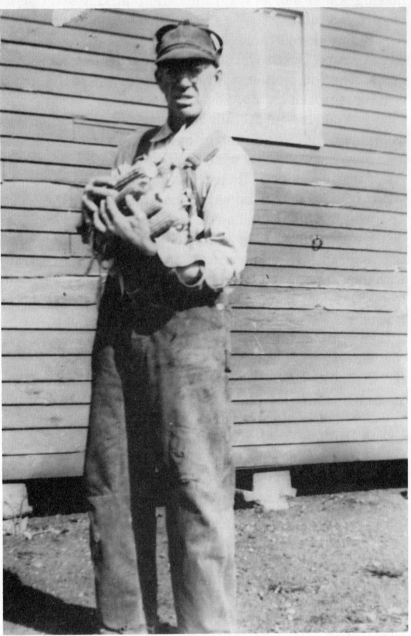

*This is my father, S. W. Harbert,
the Korn King.*

cause all the steel and factory space had been used for making war machinery. So I ended up picking sixty acres of corn by hand.

Before I was done harvesting the corn, a blizzard swept across South Dakota. The snow drifted across the fields. Then it melted a little on top of the drifts and a crust was frozen on top. South Dakota is part of the Great Plains. You can see literally for miles and miles. Montana calls itself Big Sky Country, but Big Sky fits South Dakota just as well. The wind whips across the plains and lays flat everything in its path. When a blizzard comes, all you can see is snow and sky. There are two colors: white and white. And that's how it was that year.

I was trying to harvest corn while stepping on snow that had an icy, sharp crust. I broke through the crust with every step, and fell through to my knees. Then I had to pull my foot back out, always working against the ice. Each step was painful. Soon it became clear that it wasn't a temporary condition—my knees kept on aching after the harvest was over. This was my first attack of arthritis. That was the beginning of my battle, over forty-two years ago, in 1945.

My dad also had arthritis. So he knew what was wrong. He told me it was something you just had to put up with. I knew a little bit about it. I knew it hurt. I knew that the kind we had was generally known as the *wear and tear disease, osteoarthritis*. The cartilage in the joints breaks down and then the joints hurt and start to stiffen up. About 7 percent of all people in the United States have osteoarthritis. Many people who do such heavy manual labor as farm work get this disease sooner or later.

Osteoarthritis is not precisely the same as *rheumatoid arthritis*. *Rheumatoid arthritis* starts out with a painful swelling or inflammation in the joints. After that, the cartilage starts to break down. So they both have the same end result—joint trouble and pain! They both hurt like the dickens. About 1 percent of people in the United States have *rheumatoid arthritis*.

There are many other diseases that are classified as arthritis. In fact, all combined forms of arthritis affect huge numbers of people in this country—probably over thirty-seven million people. My doctor told me many years later that I had more than one kind—but I don't remember which. I like to say, "Arthritis, I've got arthritis. It hurts like the dickens and it's been with me a long time."

Back in 1945, I had no sense about how long my struggle would take. I didn't know anything about how to take care of myself. I just kept working and followed my dad's example—tough it out.

The winter set in, and my arthritis got worse.

2

Hard Work and Hard Times: 1946–1949

Spring Brings Relief
to My Arthritis

When the next spring came around, 1946, my arthritis let
up for a while. I was ready to go. I loved farming. I loved
the outdoors and working for myself.

I also liked to have fun. I was interested in going out.
But it seemed like there weren't many women around. It
seemed like everyone was married or engaged. I'd been
going with a woman before the war, but she'd written me
one of those famous "Dear John" letters. So here I was,
nearly thirty years old, a bachelor farmer.

In 1947 we had the best crop in history. The Office of
Price Administration (OPA) lifted its controls and farm
prices shot up for a short time. For the first time I be-
lieved that I could support a wife. I'd met a young woman
who was as beautiful as any I'd seen in my travels. She
was talented—she could sing with the voice of an angel

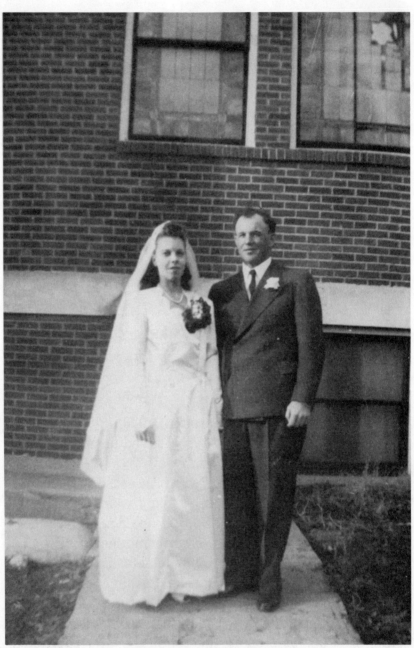

*Me and my first wife, Elaine, on our
wedding day in 1948.*

and play the piano after a fashion, although she'd had no lessons.

We got married in the fall of 1948. We didn't think about the problems ahead. Nobody knew then what was going to happen to the fate of the family farm. Nobody could've told us that economic pressures would create stress on our marriage. Nobody could foresee how bad my arthritis would become. And even if they had told us, would we have listened?

We moved into an upstairs apartment in my parents' house. We tried to adjust to the four of us living together but after a year, it was apparent that it wasn't working out. My wife and I decided we had to find another place to live.

There was a small building on the farm that wasn't being used. It was ten by sixteen feet and my father had built it so he could store their furniture, when he'd gone off to work in an airplane factory on the West Coast during the war. I scrubbed it for a week, cleaning it with disinfectant. Then I paneled the walls with hard wallboard. We moved it about fifty yards from the big house, ran wire for electricity. We set up a stove and moved in. My wife made curtains for the windows. So this became our first cozy home, the place we lived when our first baby was born.

More Harberts Home from the War

My brother came home from the navy a few years after I got out of the service. He tried to go into farming with me and my father. This arrangement lasted only a year. My brother didn't like working with my father because my father was stubborn—as I mentioned before—and opinionated. He had to have his own way. Next, my brother-in-law tried going in with us, but he and my father got along only for a year. I got along with my father. I took orders from him and did things the way he wanted. That's how we worked: He was the boss. I needed a manager: He was a pretty good one.

After a while, my father wanted to retire. He bought another piece of land. My brother was interested in keeping only the house. My arthritis was bothering me. I wondered whether a warmer climate would help me.

So, in 1949, because of all these reasons, we had a big auction to sell off the farm machinery and divide the profits.

My wife and I bought an old trailer home, which we towed to California for the winter.

California, 1949

California was no solution to my arthritis. One of my brothers, Verne, who already lived out there, got me a job setting pins in a bowling alley. Oh, did my arthritis start acting up on that job! The other pin setters would pick up a whole handful of pins at one time. I couldn't do that. I could only pick up two pins at a time, because my arthritis had progressed to my hands and wrists. I still had the arthritis in my knees, of course. The fact that I could pick up only two pins at a time meant that I had to bend over many more times than the other pin setters, and my back and knees really took a beating. I couldn't keep that job because I was too slow. Well, I figured if I couldn't do even a simple job in a bowling alley, I might as well go back to farming, which I loved. I had gone to college for two years before the war, but I hadn't received any particular training for any other kind of work.

I was disappointed that the climate in California did nothing to help my arthritis. Later in life, I heard many people tell similar stories. It's more important for us to stay home, in familiar surroundings and with people who support us, than to be in a "perfect" climate.

Homesick for the Prairies and Plains

Our adventure on the West Coast didn't turn out the way we'd hoped, all the way around. My health and our money situation saw no marked improvement. In addition, we were both homesick. We had started a family by this time and we really missed our relatives. We wanted our child to know his grandparents. We were still in love with South Dakota and its wind-swept plains.

After the winter was over, we packed up our trailer, packed up our son and packed it in—headed back home.

3

The Biggest Gamble on the Face of the Earth

Home Under the Big Sky

When we came home from California, we bought some land so we could take up farming again. I made a down payment on a quarter section of land on the Riverside corner. That's four miles east of Mitchell. You city folks probably don't know how much a quarter section is—it's one hundred sixty acres. It wasn't the greatest land. The soil was rocky and full of potholes, and Fire Steel Creek ran through it. But I liked it. We could look across the road at a little hill; it was the highest point in Hanson County. Everything else was flat. So we had a view!

I worked this farm from 1950 to 1977. They say that farming is the biggest gamble on the face of the earth. And I say that I'm the world's unluckiest gambler! For twenty-seven years, I struggled to pay for that land, raise four children, hold the family to-

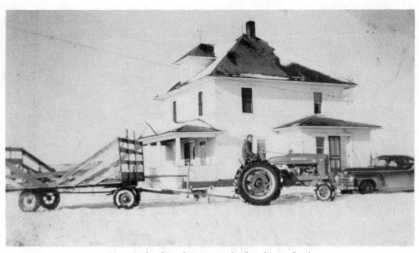

Here's the farmhouse on the land I worked from 1950 until 1977.

gether. During the twenty-seven years, my arthritis kept making bigger and bigger inroads into my life. Seldom was I without pain.

During this time, I saw the erosion of the small family farm. Farmers like me were often referred to as *lazy, little farmers*, because we had so much trouble making ends meet. I admit to being little—only five feet six in the early years—but *lazy* didn't apply. During the time I was farming, this country went through an amazing change. The family farmer was wiped out. There was an opinion out and about that the small farm was inefficient and governmental policies were geared to "ease them out of agriculture." That's a phrase I heard a lot. It was referring to people like me! I didn't want to be eased out. I had nowhere else to go.

Even though I could see the handwriting on the wall, I kept trying to make a go of it. As I said before in this story, I loved farming: working outside, being my own boss, taking care of animals. During those twenty-seven years, I almost had the land paid for three times, but some kind of financial disaster always came up—drought, hail, a medical emergency with my children, low prices.

28

Every year that I had a good crop, everyone else did, too, so the prices dropped. The years I had a bad crop, there wasn't enough money left over to pay the farm expenses. During dry years when I could farm the potholes, rain water ran off the hills and the potholes were the only place that produced a decent crop. Wet years were just the opposite. Too much water ran off the hills into the potholes, so the high ground was the only land that produced.

I tried my hand at various crops. I raised alfalfa for feed, corn for silage. I raised sheep, breeder hogs, milking cows.

When disaster hit, I would have to go to a bank to borrow money. Twice I sold off acreage for town people to "have a little acreage and build a nice home."

I was afraid to borrow money and expand the farm because my father had gone bankrupt twice that I remembered and once before I was born. This made me determined to try to pay my way as I went along. I tried to be honest, like my mother. She passed honesty on to me. I simply couldn't lie to the banker and tell him I had more collateral than really existed, even though I knew one farmer who had livestock and machinery mortgaged in two different banks, all as the same collateral.

But my experiences on the farm taught me something about judging other people. Because some people said I was lazy and I knew I was a hard worker, I decided not to criticize people and jump to conclusions about their characters. I don't judge other people. It's impossible to know the odds that others are struggling with—their money, health, stress levels.

Laughter Turns Bad Luck
Inside Out

I've been blessed with the gift of laughter. I look back at my adventures on the farm and all I can do is laugh. I laugh when I remember my jeep. When we came back from California and made the down payment on the farm, there wasn't much money left to buy livestock and machinery. I remembered how the jeep was the workhorse of the army. A person could go anywhere with it and do almost anything. So I bought one. It was an unconventional piece of farm equipment—but it worked. I used my jeep to pull old horse-drawn machinery that I could pick up for a song, because everyone else was using tractors. I plowed, disked, and dragged with the jeep. At harvest time, I bought an old combine and pulled it with the jeep. At corn-picking time, I got an old International corn picker and pulled it with my jeep. It looked goofy but it worked!

My Growing Family

By the early 1950s, my wife and I had four children— Tim, Bruce, Marta, and Mary. They were darling children. I did as much as I could to help take care of them. I washed diapers, changed diapers. On Sundays, I used to make pancakes for everybody. I made the pancakes to look like animals, with heads and tails and legs. The children loved these and would stand by the stove to request a pig or cat. I would put fruit in the batter and make syrup out of brown sugar and maple flavor. I was determined to give my children all the love I could in hopes it would take the place of the shortage of money.

During the years that our children were little, my arthritis was with me all the time. Sometimes it would come in my wrists, sometimes in my knees. It would get worse in the winter, and better in the spring and summer. But, as I said before, I was seldom without pain. Maybe I was so delighted with my children and the simple pleasures of life that I didn't pay much attention to it.

But, gradually, economic pressures wore me down, both physically and emotionally. I realized I had to find another job to support us and the farm.

4

Mink Mama, Sand Man, Salesman, Trucker

I Look for a New Way to Support My Farm Habit

My first extra job was working at the mink ranch down the road, on the way into town. I was the Mink Mama! I'll tell you what that means. I took care of the minks in their pens. I fed them and watered them. I cleaned their pens and put clean bedding in. I checked on the babies constantly—when they're born, they're only about one inch long and they can fall through the wire screen. They stay with their mothers until they're half grown. Then I would have to separate them and put them in their own pens, because they start fighting with each other. That was a tough job; they are vicious little creatures.

Every spring we had the pelting season. It was my job, along with the other workers, to kill them and skin them—we called that *fleshing*. We had to kill them with our hands to break their necks fast. It was brutal. Nowadays, I hear they use a drug to kill them fast. But back then we used our bare hands. Then we had to clean the pelts and scrape the fat off. The smell was vile. If women who want to wear mink coats could only smell that fat, they might think twice! And I have to laugh when I see TV commercials for beauty products with mink oil. That stuff really stinks! We had barrels and barrels of it.

I worked at the mink ranch for ten hours a day, six days a week, and every third Sunday. I did my farming at night and on Sundays. At the time, I had milking cows on my farm. I was milking twenty cows in the morning, before I had to be to work at 7 A.M. I worked until 6 P.M., came home to my own chores. I kept this up for nine years.

After a while at the mink ranch, arthritis seemed to be moving into my back. It was definitely getting worse. I was concerned about my health, but the economics of my life demanded that I keep working. I followed my dad's lead and just put up with it. I had trouble at night: The pain from my arthritis and from my war wound would wake me up. During the Battle of the Bulge, a fragment of a mortar shell had severed a nerve in my leg. The nerve didn't grow back together correctly. It would start twitching in the middle of the night, and numbness and pain shot up my leg.

My wife and I started having serious problems getting along. Looking back I can see that my work and my poor health took a toll on my ability to be a good husband. I was working too much to take her out dancing and do those other fun things that keep a marriage going. I can see that now. But what I thought then was that things would get better, any day. I was an optimist—always!

The Rural Economy Offers
Me a Choice

After nine years on the mink ranch, I tried to find a job that would be easier on my back. I tried many kinds of jobs, all of them associated in some way with farming.

My first job after the mink ranch was at a ready-mix cement plant. I was the sand man. I had to push a gondola-type boxcar over the pit, shovel sand out of the bottom, then run up a fifty-foot catwalk to check if the bin in the elevator was full—then run back down and move a different car over the pit. I ran up and down the catwalk, climbed onto a big tractor to move the cars, climbed in and out of the boxcars at least fifty times a day.

By fall, when the plant closed, my knees were so stiff, I could barely shuffle around. We were laid off for the winter. I could've drawn workmen's compensation but I wasn't satisfied with the forty dollars per month, so I went back to the mink ranch. Once again my old boss was good to me. He took me back and allowed me to shuffle around while we graded the mink and went through the pelting season again. I worked there for that winter and the following summer. Then arthritis got into my back, and it came back with a vengeance in my shoulder.

I started considering doing something that wouldn't require manual labor. Why not sales? A friend of mine knew about a company that wanted more sales representatives. It was a company that sold household products door-to-door. I decided to give it a try. After about three years of part-time sales, I had to conclude that I was not a born salesman. My basic honesty prevented me from hyping the products. I couldn't make customers believe they should pay the exhorbitant prices for things that were only a little better than what could be bought in a store for less. My territory was in a rural area and the pinch on the family farm was getting worse and worse. I couldn't con my neighbors!

I saw so much poverty while I was on the road, I got interested in working for the NFO, the National Farmers Organization. This group was trying to get farmers to organize to sell together and bargain for fair price contracts, the same as labor was doing so successfully for other workers. So I ended up going on the road for the NFO for a few years. This was easy on my arthritis. But it was a hard job. Farmers are an independent group. Most are probably as stubborn as I am! It's hard to get them to go together on anything. I found out that every farmer thought he was the best manager and hardest worker in America. I felt like I was knocking my head against a brick wall, trying to get such independent people to cooperate with each other, so I ended up quitting.

Oh, I tried other jobs. I worked highway construction. That's probably worse than farmwork for arthritis. I worked in two livestock sale barns. I drove a truck for a pet food plant. You name it, if it's in the country, I tried it. I tried all the choices my hometown had to offer. But as the years went by, my arthritis got so bad, I couldn't walk very well at all. I couldn't sleep at night. I took aspirin tablets every four hours, day and night. If two tablets didn't kill the pain, I took four. All those aspirins ruined my stomach. I had gas pains in my upper chest. I used every brand of antacid known.

I kept going, but I was losing hope. My marriage was falling apart but I didn't believe in divorce. I knew that broken homes were hard on children, and I didn't want to put them through that traumatic experience. I knew that in the eyes of the world, I was a failure—a lazy farmer, who could barely get by.

5

1958: Looking at Partial Disability and War Wounds

I Take My Dad's Advice and Take My Arthritis Seriously

My dad had struggled with arthritis all his life. Like many farmers, he thought his disease was a result of all the heavy work he'd done, the wear and tear on his body. His attitude was to tough it out.

But somewhere along the way, he changed his mind somewhat. In 1958, he told me I ought to go to the Veterans Administration (VA) and ask for help. He was looking out for me. Like most parents, he wanted life to be better for his children than it had been for him.

I knew that the mortar shelling and the knee injury were part of my problem. That was clear. My arthritis had started in my knees and spread to my other joints. The nerves in my legs where I had taken the mortar hit were often giving me trouble. So I went to the VA and asked about disability compensation. I had to let go of some of my pride and ask for help.

I saw a VA service officer in Mitchell. He gave me a form to fill out. I sent it to the VA hospital in Sioux Falls. A month later, I went there for an examination. I shuffled from room to room, talked to a social worker, a representative of a veteran organization, took a thorough physical examination and two doctors examined my war wounds.

The first doctor was pretty young. He had me place my foot in the middle of his chest and push. I was afraid of hurting my arthritic knee and I didn't push hard at all. He concluded that I was strong as a bull and psychosomatic.

The second doctor was older and more kindly. He examined the numb streak that went down my leg, from my calf to my big toe. It was always numb and my big toe got cold in the winter. He pricked my skin with pins to trace the numbness down my leg. He measured the calves of both my legs—one was smaller than the other. He said that was indeed a result of my wounds. He had me walk backward and forward on my toes and heels. I dragged one foot and tipped over sideways when I tried to walk on my heels. He said that was proof that my left leg was weaker.

He made a favorable report and two months later I started to receive 30 percent disability compensation from the Veterans Administration. At that time, the check was $37.50 per month. That may not sound like much now, but many times in the next twenty years, the money we got from the VA was all that kept my family fed.

Being classified as disabled also made me eligible for free hospital care. I have used the VA hospital so many times in the last few years, I'd be on welfare if I'd had to pay those bills myself. I owe a debt of gratitude to that kindly old doctor who took the time to listen to me and examine me.

The Trip to the
VA Brings Back Memories
of War

I had put all my memories of war out of my mind. But
that young doctor who called me a psychosomatic made
me so mad, all those memories came flooding back. The
idea that somebody would go off to war and be wounded
and then be called a psychosomatic was infuriating.

There's no point in pretending I hadn't been
wounded, just because I didn't apply for disability in
1945. I learned that I had to take these injuries seriously,
for they were making my arthritis worse.

My first injury was the one to my knee, and the second one was from mortar shelling. Now I'd like to tell
about how I got them both.

I was drafted in 1942. A paratrooper officer came to
basic training camp. He said that paratroopers got fifty
dollars per month extra pay for jumping out of airplanes.
I didn't consider myself to be braver than anyone else.
But I came from such a poor family that the fifty dollars
looked like a fortune. As long as you are going to get shot
at, you might as well get the extra pay. That's the way I
reasoned.

So I signed up for jump school. Then the exercise
really started. The first week we exercised eight hours a
day. It turned a short little fat farm boy into a tough
fighting man.

During my third week at jump school, training to be
a paratrooper, we were jumping off towers a hundred-
fifty feet high. We would be pulled up to the top of the
tower by a cable and our parachutes would already be
open on the way up. When we hit the top of the tower,
the chute would be released and we would float to the
ground. On one practice jump, the wind caught my parachute and blew me back up, then brought me down like

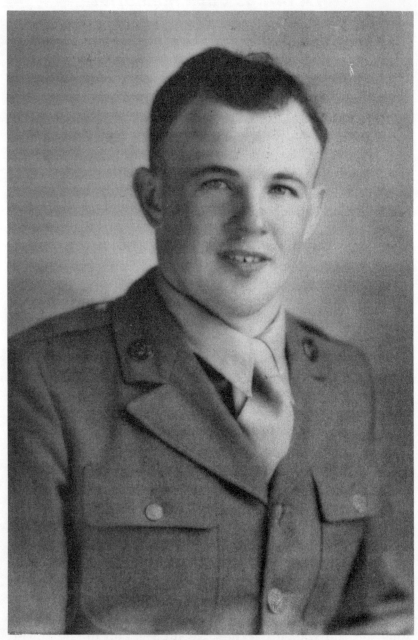

*I was 26 and in basic training at Camp Walters,
Texas, in 1942 when this picture was taken.*

the pendulum on a clock. My feet hit the ground as if I didn't even have a chute on at all. What a drop! But I must have had the luck of the Irish—from my mother— because I didn't break my back like some of the other guys. I only sprained my ankle and twisted my knee. I thought I would be OK. But three years later, arthritis hit me in the knees.

I received my second injury during the Battle of the Bulge. We were supposed to travel through the woods, parallel to a hard-surface road, and clear the enemy out of the woods in order to protect the tanks that were moving up the road. While we were doing this job, some mortar shells came in. I don't think they could see the highway, but they could hear the tanks, and aimed at the sound. The mortar shells fell short and hit us. I always say, "They didn't mean us any harm, they were shooting at the tanks!" The mortar shell landed at the feet of the lieutenant who was walking behind me. Mortar shells have grooves in them, so that they break in forty even pieces. Three of those pieces hit me from behind. In the movies, you see actors who are shot stagger around for a time, perhaps getting off a few shots of their own before they fall. Not so in real life. I was thrown to the ground with such a force that it knocked the wind out of me.

When I regained my senses, I pulled myself over to a fallen log for protection. Shells were falling all around. I yelled for a medic. I could see the lieutenant still lying where he had fallen. I think a foot was blown off because one boot was off to the side. When the medic came, I told him to go to the lieutenant first. The medic gave me a shot of morphine to kill the pain. They loaded me on a jeep and took me to the first-aid station.

That was the end of the Battle of the Bulge for me. Later the next morning, they took me to a field hospital and operated, taking two shell fragments from my right buttock and the small of my back and one from the calf of my left leg. When I woke up, the fragments were taped

41

to my wrist. The nurse asked me if I wanted to keep them for souvenirs. I declined. They were gruesome, covered with dry blood. And so I was sent to another hospital for recuperation.

What I want people to learn from my story is this: Take your injuries seriously. Take care of yourself. There are things I could've done to take care of myself but I didn't know that back then. Now I'm taking care of myself. I'm taking the time to do a good job of it, too.

6

My Last Two Jobs: Early Retirement

My Arthritis Goes Out of Control

In the 1970s, I had a job truck-driving for a pet food company. My arthritis got so bad that my boss took me off the truck. I had been loading and unloading the truck, putting boxes in the freezer. As you might imagine, working in a freezer is not a good idea for people with arthritis. It was cold and damp in there.

My boss was very kind to me and offered me another way to work. He gave me a job working with setting up the boxes that contained the beef by-products. I had to bend flat cardboard into the shape of a box and staple the corners. The boxes were flat when they came to us. By this time, arthritis was in all my joints, all the time. It had crept into my wrists and the joints of my thumbs. My fingers got stiff when I worked. I got so that I couldn't keep up bending the boxes. It hurt too bad.

I was worried about getting fired. If you're fired in

South Dakota, you can't get workmen's compensation. My boss was kind to me, again. Instead of firing me, he laid me off so I could get unemployment insurance. But this was limited to a certain amount. If I got a job for part-time work, they would subtract my pay from the weekly unemployment insurance check.

I got a job as a night janitor at a grocery store. I was able to stretch the insurance over a year that way. On that job, I had three hours to get the store cleaned, all the aisles mopped and waxed. My boss at that job was also kind to me. He knew I was walking too slowly to get all the work done, but he kept me on.

But I had trouble with my boss's supervisor. He came on inspection from Sioux Falls and noticed that some sticker price tags were stuck to the floor. He put a pencil mark on the tags, in the same way that the police sometimes put chalk on tires to see if people are staying at meters too long. I couldn't get all the sticker price tags off of the floor that next night on the job. When the supervisor came back the next day, the same stickers were still on the floor. He told the manager to fire me.

So this was the second job I had lost because I couldn't do the work. I realized my arthritis was out of control. I could no longer hold down a job.

California, Again

In order to apply for total disability status from Social Security, you have to lose two jobs and be unemployed for five months. I figured I had now done the first part—I'd been fired twice! I wondered what to do with the waiting period. I sold all my hogs. I paid the feed bills and my loan at the bank. I had no money left. I had a good car. My children, now grown, lived out in California and offered to pay for the gas if I came out to visit. I went to California, again. My relatives were wonderful hosts and took me all over but I was not active. I was sitting, sitting, and visiting—sitting in a car, sight-seeing. We had a good time, but I was doing nothing. And when you sit around doing nothing and you have arthritis, it really gets bad. Palm Springs, Disneyland, the Redwood Forest were beautiful places but they did not have what I needed to start on the road to recovery.

7

My Total Disability: When You Hit Bottom, the Only Way to Go Is Up

I Apply for Total Disability

When I came home from California in 1977, my arthritis was so bad, I was hobbling around with a cane. I couldn't bend over, or lift my arms, or raise a fork or glass to my mouth. It was time for me to apply for total disability. The Social Security people sent me to Sioux Falls to see the doctor. When the doctor examined me, he tested my arm by lifting it up, to see how high it would go. It hurt so much I thought my arm was going to break off. He also took X-rays of all my joints. Yes, he agreed. I had arthritis. He turned his report in to Social Security. I was totally disabled.

I was sixty when I applied for total disability. I was sixty-one when I got my first check.

I Go to the VA Hospital
for Help

When I took my trip to Sioux Falls to see about my disability, I decided to go to the VA hospital to find out what they could do for me. I signed in and stayed in the orthopedic ward for a week. They told me about my choices. They said I could have surgery for joint replacements, or I could try heat treatments and exercise.

I took my time thinking over these choices. It was hard for me to imagine how exercise could help me—after all, hadn't I been exercising all my life, working on the farm, working all those part-time jobs? That was my line of thinking. What I didn't know then was that all that hard work was too stressful on my joints, in contrast to slow and rhythmic exercise that doesn't stress the joints.

I thought about getting the operations. I'd had arthritis so long, it seemed like all my joints needed work. The doctor said that an operation on my knees wouldn't be so bad, but an operation on my shoulder would be harder. In my ward, there was a veteran with his leg cut off at the knee. He'd gotten an infection in his artificial hip. He swung his leg around sideways all the time when he walked. I knew that for some people the artifical joints were miracles but I just didn't feel ready.

While I was talking to the other men in the ward about surgery, I was also undergoing physical therapy every day. I did light exercise and sat in a hot whirlpool for six minutes. The hot whirlpool seemed to help a little. That little bit was enough to give me the hope that I could fight back if I could only get the energy to try.

So I made the decision to postpone surgery. I decided to go home and see what I could do.

Back at Home,
I Experience Severe
Depression

Even though I knew I had made the right decision for me, when I left the VA hospital and returned home, I was severely depressed. I was still living out on the farm, but my wife was no longer living with me. I knew it was just a matter of time before we did the paperwork for a divorce. I didn't want to face it. I looked out the window and saw the farm that I had loved for all of my adult life. My marriage was gone, my farm was in danger. I said to myself, "I guess I never got the hang of it." At that time I thought of myself as a loser—now I prefer to say that the Good Lord never intended for me to have money. He had other plans for me.

At the age of sixty-one, I faced the prospect of not only being miserable, but the prospect of being miserable for a long time. Because all the men in my family lived well into their nineties. I was only sixty-one! I had definitely hit bottom. I had never been so depressed. I had to face living with a chronic illness that has no cure. I think that just hearing the words *chronic illness* are enough to get a person down.

I admit that at that time, I even cried—tears would come into my eyes for no reason. My pride and self-respect were gone. My initiative was gone. My fighting, never-say-die spirit lay dormant within me. My brain was numb. I even considered suicide. Later, several years later, I found out that this kind of depression is not unusual for seniors. Seniors have the second highest suicide rate of any age group. Teenagers are first.

It looked to me like my arthritis had won the thirty-year-old battle we had been fighting.

The Spark of Life

But after I sat around for a while, watching those stupid soap operas, I couldn't stand it. My inactivity was driving me crazy. My dislike of inactivity won out over the depression! Somewhere deep within me, there was a spark of my former self. I've heard it said that there is a spark of God within each of us. Perhaps it was that spark that came to life and gave me the courage to try again.

Or maybe the spark was another word for the stubbornness in me. I inherited this from my Welsh father: just plain stubbornness. As I said earlier in my story, the Harberts have a stubborn streak a mile wide. It's true. I decided to get up out of my chair and try the remedy the doctors ordered—exercise.

I Start Walking the Road to Recovery

The road to recovery was the county road that ran by my farm. I got up and started walking it every day. I had to use my cane. Walking was painful. I headed out for the country school where my children had gone. It was three quarters of a mile to the school. Then I would turn around and head back home. I couldn't walk fast. I got tired before I could finish that final stretch.

Anna Uhrich Offers Me a Ride and Changes My Life

Sometimes neighbors stopped to offer me a ride. My neighbors were friendly country people I'd known for many years. I knew all the kids. We had all helped each other out when our kids were little. I had been the 4-H leader.

One of these neighbors was Anna Uhrich. She stopped one day and said, "Virgil, what is it you're doing walking down this country road every day?"

"My arthritis got the best of me," I said, "But I'm not going to let it get me down."

"I've noticed you," she said. "You've been walking faster. I was wondering if you'd consider doing me a favor."

Anna didn't even have to ask if I'd consider doing her a favor. I would do almost anything for that woman. She'd been a friend of mine and my family's for many years. She and her husband lived down the country road by the school and I lived by the road to town. Sometimes my kids would go to her house after school and she welcomed them, even though she had ten kids of her own. If there was a blizzard, she and her husband would ride their snowmobile to my farm and then take their pickup to town to their jobs. They'd come back at night and park the pickup in my driveway, and snowmobile home over the road that hadn't been plowed yet. It is pretty wild out here when the blizzards hit.

So of course I said without any hesitation, "Of course, I'll do a favor for you, Anna. What is it?"

"Well, Virgil, we've been having some square dances at the Senior Center. There's lots of widows who come— but a definite shortage of men. Last time we had twenty women and four men! Would you consider helping us out?"

I smiled at her and replied, "I'd be glad to help you out, Anna. But I can barely walk. I'm not sure how dancing will go!"

Little did I know that by helping her out I was going to help myself to a new way of life. Square dancing was going to show me a new direction for my battle against arthritis. It was going to show me the way to recovery.

51

As you might imagine, I hadn't been going out much. When people are depressed, they don't even think about going out. That was true for me. I was having all kinds of fears, too. I didn't trust myself to drive after dark because I was so slow getting my foot on the brakes. My oldest son offered to drive me to the dance. And so we set off. My first night out in months.

Since my son drove me, he figured he might as well join in. So they had two extra men for dancing. I had never square danced in my life but the caller was good. He would take us through the sets slowly and show us what each call meant.

Everyone had a good time because everyone could figure out how to do it. We kept coming back. Some of us would forget the dances from one week to the next and we had to learn all over again. What a memory some of us have! The caller was patient with us and taught us over and over each week. I got so I could shuffle around quite well. My knees were getting limbered up. Dancing was more fun than walking along a road by myself. I started to feel some hope for myself. I was making new friends.

Square dancing gave me hope. What I thought was my stubbornness gradually changed to the secret ingredient of happy living—hope!

I had undying gratitude to Anna Uhrich. I hoped I would be able to repay her some day. If it hadn't been for her, I think right now I'd be in an old soldiers' home—sitting in a wheelchair.

8

I Do-si-do
My Way to Exercise
Class

Square Dancing
Loosens Up My Body and
My Attitude

All that square dancing got me limbered up. My knees got limbered up. Getting out and seeing people got me out of my misery and self-pity. I had something to look forward to for the first time in several years.

All of a sudden, it seemed like there were lots of things I could do to get healthier. Maybe those things had been there all along and I just couldn't see them when I was depressed.

After several months I realized that I could stop using my cane! I was so much better I didn't need it any more.

Wake Up and Smell the Coffee: Put Hope into Action

Arthritis is a chronic illness. There just isn't going to be a cure in my lifetime. At least that's how I need to look at it. It is necessary for me to accept my arthritis as something that's going to be with me from now on. I pray for a cure. But I can't live *hoping* for one. What I have to *hope for* is that I can live with my arthritis. I can have a good life.

I decided it was up to me to take charge of my arthritis. I decided to see what else I could do to take care of myself. Square dancing was a big step, but I couldn't stop there. I wanted more. I wanted to get better.

I'd really loved the hot whirlpool at the VA hospital. Anna told me there was an exercise class at the local YMCA. She said that anyone who went to the class could use the hot whirlpool at the Y. I hadn't even known there was a whirlpool in Mitchell! So I started going to the Y for both exercising and the whirlpool. I started going in 1977 and I'm still going to this day, 1988.

When I went to the exercise class, the exercises were so painful that I knew I had to look around for some way to deal with my pain.

Temporary Relief, Hope, and False Cures

I had made so much improvement with the square dancing, that I knew I was on the right track. But doing exercise really hurt. I wanted some relief, even temporarily. I was taking the maximum amount of aspirin.

Some people can find some relief with prescription drugs, from their doctors, but I didn't want to deal with all the side effects. I looked for other solutions.

People were always telling me about remedies. One was to take a mixture of honey and lemon juice three times a day. Another was to wear a brass bracelet around your arm. I got ticked off at their advice. Some people just can't accept the fact that there is *no cure* for arthritis.

I also got ticked off at the commercials on TV. The ones that say a pill will bring fast relief for the *"minor pains of arthritis."* The person who wrote that obviously never had arthritis. The pains of arthritis aren't *"minor."* When I was wounded during the Battle of the Bulge and the shell fragments threw me to the ground, it wasn't nearly as bad as the constant grating pain that accompanied every step I took for so many years while farming and working my other jobs.

In my search of freedom from pain, I decided to go to the hot whirlpool every day. That worked wonders. It was the most reliable activity for dealing with pain. I've heard that people in other cities also love hot whirlpools. I heard one woman say, "God bless the pool."

For a while, I tried acupuncture treatments. I don't know if they would help everybody, but they helped me. I heard about acupuncture from my sister-in-law, who has arthritis, too. She lives north of the dam that forms Lake Oahe, north of Pierre, South Dakota. Her fingers were all gnarled and she could barely walk around her kitchen to fix a meal. She started going to a chiropractor, who gave her acupuncture treatments. She'd gotten so much better, she said, she could "jump around like a spring chicken."

I gave it a try. It turned out to be wonderful temporary relief of my pain. Again, I need to say that it wasn't a cure. It was temporary. What the acupuncturist does is stick very fine needles in the nerve centers. The pins block the nerves for a while so your brain doesn't get the message that it hurts. I went out there for ten treatments, spread out over three and a half days. I didn't have the money to stay in a motel room, so I fixed up the back seat of my car so I could sleep there.

The acupunture treatments helped alleviate my pain for about four months after each treatment. I went back about every six months, and the treatments helped me be able to start exercising.

All in all, I went for acupuncture treatments for three years. After that, I was well enough to do without them.

Exercise Class
Becomes a Way of Life

With the help of square dancing, hot whirlpool, and acupuncture, I was able to take part in the exercise class at the Y. At first, I could hardly do any of the exercises. I moved slowly, but I kept going. The leader of the class when I started was a woman named Ruth Bateman. She taught exercises that she'd gotten from a doctor. Eventually she wanted to spend time with her children in Florida and she found us a new teacher: Alma Summers, who was wonderful in the way she encouraged all of us to keep trying. Keep stretching! Keep flexing!

After a year and a half of the class, I was finally able to do all the exercises. My joints had become flexible, my muscles were stronger. But it was a long struggle. I'm grateful to all the kind people who encouraged me along the way: Ruth, Alma, and all the people in the class.

At the end of a year and a half, I was ready to go! Square dancing was great, now I was ready to go out dancing to country-western music. I felt OK about driving a car.

I thought I knew the direction my life was taking—better health, mobility, vim, and vigor, a positive attitude, and fun! That was all true—but there were many more wonderful things in store for me. Life remained unpredictable—even for a man who was sixty-five years old.

9

Stress, Relaxation, and Letting Go

I Let Go of the Farm and Move into Town

After taking charge of my arthritis by walking the country road to recovery and starting to learn to exercise properly, my life changed fast. I can't even keep track of what happened when. As I started to improve with all my stretching and flexing, I realized that it was time to leave my farm. That part of my life was over. Once I accepted my chronic illness, took charge of it, instead of letting it run me, it was easier to let go of the farm.

I heard somebody say that nothing new can come into your life until you let go of the old.

I moved into an apartment in Mitchell. Soon after that, the farm was turned over to my wife as part of our divorce settlement.

I Look for
Ways to Relax and
Find Support

All of us with arthritis know that emotional stress can cause a flare-up of the illness. Emotional stress does not *cause* our illness but it seems to aggravate it. When I look back on all those years on the farm, it seems the economic stress and marital discord took a toll on my feelings and my body. When I started to improve, it was important for me to find ways to relax. I had to make a schedule. I had to make sure that I did something relaxing every day.

I started going out more on weekends. I liked to go dancing at the VFW. This get-together involved dancing to country music. I know how to waltz and do other fancy steps but I don't like them as well as dancing to good country music—I can just relax and move any way I want. That's fun for me and good for my arthritis. Following the waltz tends to make me cramp up.

I could see that it was good for me to get out and socialize. People need people. I could see that this socializing was helping me deal with my pain and my disability, just as much as the socializing I did with my friends in the exercise class at the Y. I learned that this kind of support really helps. What I've noticed since then is that support is crucial for everyone with a chronic illness. It's important to have lots of people you can talk to. It's dangerous to keep your feelings shut up inside. Now, I happened to like to go dancing. Dancing's not for everyone. But *everyone* with a chronic illness needs to get out of the house and talk to other people.

In the bigger cities, there are now groups called *support groups* for people with arthritis. What a great idea! We don't have a group called a support group in Mitchell, but I like to think of my exercise group as a place where people do get support from each other. When I hear everyone laughing and talking about their ailments *and* their accomplishments, I know people are giving to each other. I just read an article about some new research that says that people with rheumatoid arthritis who go to a support group have less pain and tenderness in their joints than people who don't go to a group. So I think everybody should find some kind of group—get out of your house or your apartment and find an exercise group, a support group, a hot whirlpool, or a friend! If there's no group in your town, find someone else who has arthritis and make a date to get together for coffee once a week.

The Arthritis Foundation is a nationwide organization that can give you information about the disease and about support groups. Here is the national address. (You can check your phone book to see if there's a local chapter.)

ARTHRITIS FOUNDATION
1314 Spring Street, N.W.
Atlanta, Georgia 30309
(404) 872-7100

Relaxing with Hobbies

As I said earlier, I think it was my dislike of inactivity that won out over my depression. Part of my recovery was figuring out what to do with all the time available in retirement. Sure, I was busy with the whirlpool and exercise but I still had time on my hands. I'm not the sort of person who likes to sit around. I've got energy to burn. Even today, after I work out at the Y, sit in the whirlpool, go to my part-time job, I still have energy to burn. If I stay inside I start brooding and I can feel myself going down, depressed. I feel lonely. A penned-up animal. I want out.

From what I've seen, there are lots of people who

don't know what to do with all the free time on their hands in retirement. So I thought I'd tell you the story of one of my hobbies.

When I was out in California, right before I applied for my total disability status, my brother took me through the Redwood National Park. We stopped at a souvenir shop and saw some beautiful coffee tables. They were made from cross sections of giant redwood trees, stained dark mahogany, and polished like glass. I thought that maybe I could take up woodworking and take my mind off my arthritis. I might be able to do sanding and finishing, as long as I didn't have to reach my arms up over my head. I could sit down and do it. I had always been handy.

So when I got home from California in 1977, I looked around for a project. I thought of using old barn wood to make tables and picture frames. The old barn on my farm had blown down recently. It was almost down in 1950 when I bought the place. I had braced up the sagging roof with poles and had used it for many years. It had never been painted. The old drop siding was weather-beaten and cracked from so many years of neglect. I found that most of the old barns had blown down, or their roofs had caved in and the farmers had bulldozed them into piles and burned them. So there wasn't much drop siding left in the country. The barns had been replaced by steel sheds. This gave drop siding a nostalgic flavor. Lumber companies didn't even make it any more.

So I took up antique wood projects. I bought a table saw and miter box at an auction and made some picture frames. I made three coffee tables from the manger from my old barn. One coffee table had a hole in it where we used to tie the horses. We would stick the halter rope through the hole.

After working on wood for a while, I got a hankering to brighten up all that old gray wood. I made a table with a picture of a horse's head painted in the center. I've never had an art lesson, but I learned! Hey, we have to keep learning! I painted a lariat around the horse's head and all around the edge of the table.

As I said earlier, I was a country music fan. You might have guessed that I love Johnny Cash. I made a table and painted a picture to illustrate his song, "Ghost Riders in the Sky." It showed an old cow-hand on a ridge watching as the devil's herd floated by with riders trying to catch them. All the steers were branded 666—that's the devil's brand. I thought that was funny.

I had so much fun taking up this hobby. It kept me busy, it took my mind off my aches and pains, and it gave me something to look forward to. If I had been doing the same amount of work with a boss looking over my shoulder, I would have been griping about all the hard work. But I didn't. This wasn't work, it was play. When I left the farm, my hobby came with me. I could go on and on about all the paintings I've done since then. But I want to just make the point how much this hobby helped me. It helped me relax, while my body was getting better. It's been a friend through many days of pain.

I think of all the people I know who are retired. We worked hard. We tried to do the right thing and support our families. Now it's time for some fun. If we don't relax and have some fun now, when will we? And if we never had time for hobbies before, what's stopping us now? Fear that we're too old to learn new hobbies? No, we're never too old.

There used to be a sign in the Senior Center that I like to say out loud:

BE PATIENT:
GOD ISN'T THROUGH WITH ME YET

10

Stretching and Flexing Lead to a New Chapter in My Life

I Meet Up with a New Romance

By now, I was feeling really positive and happy. I liked going out and being with people. I wasn't especially looking for a new romance. Dancing was fun and so was playing the field!

But along the way, I met a woman I really enjoyed being with, Leona Butterfield. I don't know what she saw in me—maybe it was my dancing, I don't know what else it could've been. Anyway, one thing led to another. I had to have a prostate operation and she helped me through that recuperation. Then she got sick and I took care of her. I think you really get to know someone when they're sick. You get to know their true self.

We both have a little trouble with our memories—as I recall our romance, we danced at the Moose Lodge, but she says she asked me to dance at the VFW at my sixty-fifth birthday party! We finally realized we wanted to get

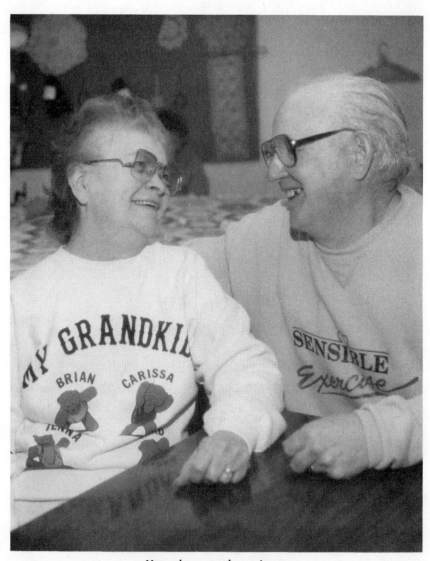

Me and my sweetheart, Leona.

married. We set the date. I joke about how I can't remember my anniversary—I have to go home and find our wedding picture and turn it over and look at the date written on the back: May 1, 1983.

We've had a good life together. We've been with each other through many changes. I don't know why people say life begins at forty. It's never too late to have a hobby—and it's never too late for a happy marriage.

And the marriage wasn't the only big change in my life in 1983.

A Fateful Turn of Events

After I was in the exercise class for about six years, our leader, Alma Summers, became ill and could no longer lead the class. She was seventy-four years old. We were all very sad about her illness. This was in 1983.

This event left our class without a leader.

Everybody wanted me to take over. I guess they liked my enthusiasm and hopefulness. I couldn't believe the turn of events. Here just a short time before I was so crippled I could barely walk. With the hot whirlpool, the acupuncture, and the exercises every day, I had made an amazing recovery. I was up and about and on the go! Sixty-seven years old and on the go!

I was excited to get up in the morning, even when my arthritis had kept me awake in the night. I even could remember being a boy and how my nickname then was "Happy." This memory no longer made me feel sad. I had regained my happy disposition.

So I said, "Sure, I'll take over." Arthritis no longer ruled my life. I had taken charge of it. I owed my recovery to many people—Alma, Ruth, Anna, the kind doctor in Sioux Falls, the staff at the Senior Center—and I thought that leading the class would be a way to pass this kindness on to others. Besides, if I was in charge of the class, I would have to show up and that meant I would be doing the exercise I needed for my own well-being!

How I Adapted the Exercise Class to My Arthritis

Because of my own illness, it was always necessary for me to move slowly, sometimes more slowly than the other people. It hurt me to go faster. So when I took over as leader, I kept the exercises at a slow pace. You may wonder where we learned the exercises. The first leader, Ruth Bateman, got some from a doctor. Then Alma added some when she took over. But we've added more and changed all of them, over the years.

The first change I made was in the counting. Alma used to always count to four. I read somewhere that exercise needed to be regular. So I decided to make the count go to twenty or forty so we could get into a slow rhythm. And I kept the rhythm slow.

Then I talked with the class members about what they wanted. I was open to the suggestions of the class. I have a close rapport with them, because we're all in the same boat. They brought in exercises that they read about or learned when they went south for the winter. If somebody wanted to try one, we tried it together, and if it worked, we added it to our routine. For example, the Dutch Windmill was brought up by a class member who spends her winters in Texas.

I Read to Learn About
Health and Recovery

I started reading everything I could find on health and exercise. I found exercises in the newspaper. Some of these we tried, and slowed them down so we could do them comfortably.

I read *The Reader's Digest* for information that I could use to give my class pep talks. I wanted to give them hope. I wanted them to keep coming back! Not sit at home feeling scared and depressed and old. In *The Reader's Digest* there were more and more articles about how exercise could delay the inroads of one disease or another. There's a long list of diseases that can be helped but not cured. One article said, "Exercise is the Fountain of Youth." The writer said that people can live from ten to fifteen years longer if they exercise. I don't know if I believe that. What I do believe is that life will be better and happier while we live if we exercise. The effects of arthritis and other diseases can be delayed.

I found several books on arthritis that could be useful to people.

One is titled *Natural Relief for Arthritis*. The publisher is Rodale Press, 1983. The author is Carol Keough; editors, Prevention Magazine.

Another good book is: *The Arthritis Helpbook: A Tested Self-Management Program for Coping with Your Arthritis*. The authors are Kate Lorig, R.N., Dr.P.H., and James F. Fries, M.D. It is published by Addison-Wesley, 1986.

I'm always on the lookout for books on this subject. But the interesting thing is—all the books always say what I discovered through my own pain—that you just have to get out there and exercise and take charge of your arthritis. Sitting around will only make it worse.

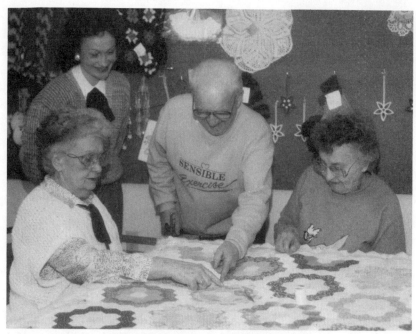

Our Senior Center has lots of action!

I Learn by Going Out to Meetings

I tried to make the class better by going out to meetings. I became active in the Health Advocacy Program of the AARP (American Association of Retired Persons). I went to health fairs to learn what I could. Now I'm not a doctor, not a physical therapist. But there were doctors and physical therapists at those health fairs and I talked with them. They told me what people *should* do and should *not* do when they're exercising. They told me how people can exercise without injury. I thought about what they told me and changed our routine accordingly. I found out that more research says that exercise *doesn't have to be fast to be effective.* I thought it was funny that my method—slow and easy and sensible exercises—would turn out to be what the current research said was good. For example, none of the people in my class would ever consider jogging. It's too much of a jolt to the joints. It's a terrible idea for people with arthritis to jog. But it took a while for research to catch up with common sense.

And people love to come to my class. After a while, it got so that my class was becoming an institution.

A New Chapter in Other People's Lives

After people took my class, many of them went on to other activities. Some of them added modified aerobic exercise to their routine—more walking, dancing. What I emphasized to people is that I will help them get started. My class is a beginning. I set it up so that many people can become active and mobile again, by stretching out their stiff muscles. I never promised anyone they would look like body-builders or TV stars. I promised people that their lives would change. And they did.

11

My Sense of Humor Gets a Workout

Me and My Jokes

I have to admit it—I love to tell jokes. I love to laugh. Leading the exercise class gave me a captive audience for my jokes. It inspired me to be on the lookout for more jokes. I started looking through the newspaper and three newsletters from veterans' organizations. I even bought a book of Norwegian jokes—*Ole and Lena.*

People got a kick out of my jokes. So I've kept them going to this day.

Usually I like to work new jokes into our routine. I save them up for the Wiggle and Close Exercise. We wiggle our fingers and then close our fists. At the end of the exercise, I say, "Shake 'em out." And we shake our hands for a minute. It's a pause in the routine. That's when I tell jokes. One woman in the class is really religious. I shouldn't say which church, because people can be religious coming from any church. She thinks my jokes are too raw. Anyway, she puts

71

her hands over her ears when I start in on a joke—but she lifts the heels of her hands up off her ears so she can hear. I can tell she is chuckling to herself.

Well, I have to watch it sometimes. But I think I do OK. I've cleaned up my act. After all, I worked my whole life with men who couldn't talk without using four-letter words. Considering that, I think I do pretty well when I talk in public.

On the other hand, some people fault me for telling risqué jokes—but we must keep our sense of humor to help us overcome our problems. Laughter is the best medicine. If I tell a so-called clean joke to my class, no one laughs. If I tell the other kind, they all laugh. It isn't that we do these things. It is just that we like to laugh about things that might have happened. And perhaps did when we were young.

So, here are some of my favorite jokes:

I didn't sleep too well last night—arthritis kept waking me. Had to make exercise class by ten. Stumbled into the bathroom, put toothpaste in my hair, washed my teeth with Brylcreem. Believe me, 'a little dab 'll do ya.'"

A lady in my exercise class walks all over town. One night she woke up screaming, "My legs have turned black." Her sister called the doctor. The doctor took off her black stockings.

A politician went to an Indian reservation to get votes. He made big promises, as politicians are prone to do. "If you Indians vote for me, I'll build a new road through here." The Indians said, "oomgla, oomgla." The politician didn't know the Indian language. He thought they were cheering. "If you Indians vote for me, I'll build a new hospital here." "Oomgla, oomgla." "If you Indians vote for me, I'll build a new school here." "Oomgla, oomgla." Then the chief stood up and said, "You are so good to us Indians, I'll give you a horse. Just go to my stable and pick out any horse you want. But be careful so you don't step in the 'oomgla.'"

Senior Citizens are accused of being forgetful. There was this old guy who could really play golf, but he couldn't see too good. He had an old friend go halfway down the fairway to watch where the ball went. He hit the ball straight down the fairway but lost track of it. He cupped his hands and shouted, "Did I hit the ball?" "Yes, you hit the ball." "Was it a good one?" "Yes, it was a good one." "Did you see where it went?" "Yes, I saw where it went." "Where did it go?" "I forgot."

I was out jogging one day. This old guy came by me like I was standing still. I said, "Hey, wait. How old are you?" "I'm eighty-five." "Eighty-five and jogging like that? Do you also have sex?" "Almost every night." "Almost every night at your age? Fantastic!" "Yep. Almost Monday, almost Tuesday, almost Wednesday."

Back in the "Dirty Thirties" they had Civilian Conservation Corps camps for girls as well as boys. Girls had to pass physical exams before they could go. One girl I heard of asked the doctor, "Can I get venereal disease by sleeping with another girl?" The doctor said, "Yes, that's the way I got mine."

During the Depression years, money was hard to come by. I asked one farmer how he got rich. "It's a long story. Put out the candle and I'll tell you."

Someone said to me, "You are in good shape for seventy-one." I said, "Longevity runs in my family. My father was a hundred and one when he married a twenty-one-year-old woman." "At that age why would he want to get married?" "Who said he wanted to?"

When I was young, I took a Norwegian girl to a dance seventy-five miles away. She was a goer. We danced all night. I was all worn out. On the way home, I got so sleepy, I just had to stop the car in a roadside park to sleep awhile. She snuggled up close to me, thinking something was going to happen—maybe I would propose. I sat with my hands on the wheel, and leaned my head back against the seat. When I went to sleep, my hand fell on her knee. She said, "Virgil, you can go furder den dat." So I started the car and drove home.

There was a little town in Minnesota that had in its charter that there must always be a Norwegian on their police force. Their Norwegian died, so they called "Ole" in. They said, "Ole, if you can answer just one question, you can be on our police force. Take your time to find the answer to this question. Who killed Abraham Lincoln?" Ole was so proud, he went strutting down the street telling everyone he was on the police force. "I've only been on the force an hour, and already they got me working on a murder mystery."

Speaking of riddles, Gracie Allen was good at making up riddles. She asked George Burns, "What's the difference between a cucumber and an umbrella?" He didn't know, so she said, "I don't know either. I just make up riddles— I don't make up the answers."

I read George Burns's book, *How to Live to be 100 or Over*. I like his attitude. He says surround yourself with beautiful women. There are about sixty-five people in my exercise class. Five of them are men. The women are fat, short, tall, skinny. They are all beautiful to me. George says he exercises everyday. If he is going to walk two blocks, he eats two prunes. If he is going to walk three blocks, he eats an extra prune for breakfast. He also says to avoid funerals—especially your own.

So many seniors actually worry themselves to death. I hate to hear them talk around our senior center. "This old friend died, that old friend died. I'm not long for this world." A local funeral parlor even brings in leftover funeral bouquets. How depressing! I have heard of an eighty-three-year-old lady in Arkansas who has a more positive approach. She says she has four boyfriends. She gets up with *Will*-power, goes for a walk with *Art*-hritis, comes home with *Charlie*-horse, and goes to bed with *Ben*-gay.

There was this minister and priest who used to ride their bikes in the park for exercise. They would meet there and make small talk. One day the minister came on foot saying, "Someone stole my bike." A week later, he had his bike back. "Did you find out who stole your bike?" the priest asked. "Well, not exactly. I went into the pulpit and started delivering a strong sermon on the Ten Commandments. When I got to 'Thou shalt not commit adultery,' I remembered where I left my bike."

I quite often go to sleep in church. I claim it's because my conscience is clear. One day the preacher thought he would embarrass me enough so that I would stay awake. He arranged with the rest of the congregation to remain seated when he said "Stand up." I was half asleep in the middle of his sermon, when I heard him say, "Stand up." What he had really said is, "Anyone who wants to go to Hell, stand up." I looked around and discovered the rest were all seated. I said, "Well I don't know exactly where, but it looks like the preacher and I are the only ones going."

A clean-living South Dakota boy who knew nothing of city ways went to school and became a priest. His first parish was in a big-city hospital. He went for a walk downtown for exercise. On a corner in front of a bar stood a hooker. "Father would you like a quicky for five dollars?" He didn't know what that was, so he declined and went back to the hospital. He asked one of the sisters, "What's a quicky?" "Five dollars—just like downtown."

Some of the ladies in my exercise class have raised large families. I heard one talking to a woman who didn't have any children. "We have been praying for children every night for ten years," she said, "but we haven't been blessed." "That isn't the way you get them," the other woman replied.

A farmer took his wife to the doctor because they didn't have children. The doctor asked, "Have you had intercourse?" "Intercourse, what's that?" the farmer asked. So the doctor put the wife on the examining table and proceeded to demonstrate. "Now if you do that Mondays, Wednesdays, and Fridays for the next month, you will have a child." "Well doctor, I can bring her in here Mondays and Tuesdays, but on Fridays I have a Farm Bureau Meeting."

All my life I've been looking for the gold at the end of the rainbow. I finally found the pot. It hangs over my belt.

If Dolly Parton was a farmer, she would be flat-busted, too.

Three men arrived at the pearly gates about the same time. Saint Peter checked his list. "How come you are here? You aren't due for several years." The man answered, "I suspected my wife was seeing another man. I came home early. There was a cigar in the ashtray, but no man. I thought I passed him in the elevator. I looked out the window—a man came out of the building, stopped on the curb to light a fresh cigar. I was so mad, I picked up the refrigerator and threw it out the window at that man. The refrigerator was so heavy, I had a heart attack." Saint Peter talked to the second man. "You are also here too early. How come?" "I don't know," the man said. "I was standing on the curb, lighting a cigar. A refrigerator fell on me." Saint Peter talked to the third. "How come you are here so soon?" "I was hiding in the refrigerator," he said.

A lady in my exercise class is a very good cook. One night she wanted to impress her friends with steaks smothered in mushrooms, but she didn't like the high price of mushrooms, and she thought they might be poisonous. So she tried them on her dog. The dog lapped them up and ran outside. The guests ate the steaks and enjoyed them. Then the kids came in. "Mama, Spot is dead!" Panic! Pump the guests' stomachs! Then the kids came back in. "Mama, the truck that ran over Spot didn't even stop."

A lady who spends her winters in Texas brought the "Texas windmills" to our exercise class. It's part of our Sensible Exercise videotape. By the way, I've been to Texas. Texas coffee is so thick it will float a spoon—if the spoon doesn't dissolve before you can stir the coffee.

I believe Ronald Reagan when he says the economy is improving. I was talking to my garbage man. He says his business is picking up.

Laughing at Our Frailties

You know, standing up in front of a group isn't the easiest thing in the world. My memory isn't the greatest. I get more addle-brained every day. It helps me to laugh at myself.

When I first started leading the class, sometimes I would forget to do one exercise. I would just plain leave it out. The great thing about my class is they always yell and holler if I forget one.

So sometimes now I just pretend to forget. See if they're paying attention! Sometimes I pretend I forgot the exercise is over and I keep counting, forty-six, forty-seven, forty-eight, forty-nine. Somebody will yell out, "Virgil, stop it, we're done at forty!"

I'm not the only one with problems with memory. It's such a common problem to us seniors that almost any situation involving memory lapse will bring out a hearty laugh

77

from everyone. For example, one day at the end of our exercise class, we started singing "Happy Birthday" to one of our dear friends in the class. Everybody did fine remembering the words to the song and the tune—but when we got to the point where we were supposed to say her name, all of us drew a blank. We had to stop the song, laugh, say, "What's your name again?" Then we continued.

I love it when people laugh. It keeps us alive. And if some of my jokes seem corny, I just say, "Well, I'm from Mitchell, South Dakota, home of the Corn Palace. What do you expect?"

Sometimes I think the reason people keep coming back to my class is to hear what *that old goof is going to say next.* But come back they do, and every week someone steps up to me to say thanks for the good exercise and the *fun.*

The Body's Natural Painkillers

Everybody knows that laughing makes us feel better, even when we're ill. Now research has found out that laughing and exercise let the body release endorphins. Endorphins are called *the body's natural painkillers.* Endorphins help relax and heal the body. They are stronger than morphine. So I figure people are getting a double dose by coming to my class—they get to exercise *and* laugh. So I say, keep on laughing. Keep on exercising. And if I can play the clown and help people get better, why not?

12

Mitchell's Exercise Guru

My Class Is a Hit

I took over the exercise class because I thought I could be of service to others. I had no idea that it would be a hit. More and more people started coming and enjoying my class.

I'm not the only one whose life changed dramatically. I observed other people going through some amazing changes after they had been exercising for some time. First I saw a change in the so-called "frozen joints," the immobility and stiffness. Then there was a change in attitude. It's a mystery how it works. Maybe it's those endorphins, the natural painkillers. But whatever the reason, people who took my class experienced a change in attitude for the better.

Once optimism takes over, who knows what will happen next! Some people found the energy to get their weight under control. Others started in on new hobbies. Everyone just perked up and enjoyed life more.

I believe now that I can promise anyone that their life will be better if they start exercising—I can't predict *how* it will be better but I know it will be better.

After a while, we named the class: Sensible Exercise. We started having the class in the Mitchell Senior Center, three times a week.

The Media Come Calling

People around town started talking about all these seniors getting out and getting in shape. A reporter even came from Sioux Falls to Mitchell to write up a story about our class.

Well, in this article, which was published in the *Sioux Falls Argus Leader*, the reporter called me Mitchell's Exercise Guru. When I first read the article, I felt insulted. A picture flashed in my mind of a person with a long beard and a long, flowing robe who was deported because he didn't pay his taxes. But then I looked up the word *guru* in the dictionary. It said that a guru is a teacher. Well, that's what I am. I'm a teacher. I teach exercise. I preach exercise.

I want people to follow my example and get out and exercise. Any one can do it, all you have to do is try. What I say to people is, "If a totally disabled man could try, so can you. I can't guarantee that anyone will live longer, but I can guarantee that you will live a happier life, while you are living, because exercise doesn't affect just the body—it affects the mind. It makes you feel better about yourself."

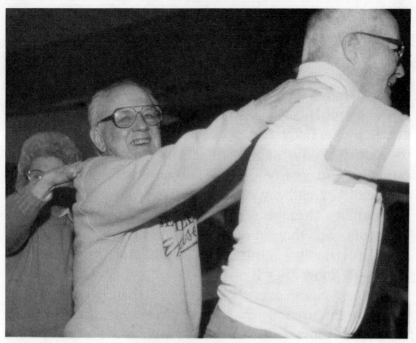

*This is our favorite part of
exercising—getting a neck rub!*

What's Different About
My Exercise Class

I've already explained that my humor gets a workout
while I'm leading my class. It's pretty obvious that I love
that part of my class.

But I get a kick out of other aspects of working with
my people. For one thing, people show up for my class
wearing all kinds of clothes. Nobody is competing for the
fanciest exercise suit. I tell people, "Wear comfortable,
warm clothes. Wear shoes and socks." I get great clothes
at the Salvation Army. Well, people just walk in—wearing whatever. One of the fellows comes in his suit. He
takes off the jacket, but not the tie. Because we do our
stretching and bending and loosening up either standing
up or on a chair, there's no problem with people getting
their street clothes dirty on the floor. And we don't need
shiny tights! That's for the young people who are still try-

ing to look sexy. We're beyond that now, trying to look a certain way. Not that we're over the hill!

My class is a beginning class. If people really want to get in shape after they've worked with me for a while, they can move on to fancy workout clothes. Go over to the fitness gym! But since we're all beginners, nobody laughs at what somebody can or can't do. We each just do what we can. Nobody makes fun of anybody. The point is to compete with yourself. Each person is stretching for better health. I call myself a beginner, because I regained my mobility through sensible exercise. But I have to begin again each day, in order to maintain my range of motion. If I don't exercise, my joints start to creak and groan—I know they'll stiffen up on me.

In my class, everybody goes at their own speed. If people want to stop, they stop. If they need to do very, very small movements in the beginning, then that's what they do.

I Learn More About Arthritis: Osteoporosis

After I was doing the class for a while, I got interested in learning about osteoporosis. I was volunteering then for the AARP Health Advocacy Program.

I went to some informational meetings and learned that osteoporosis is a weakening of the bones. Some people call it "brittle bones." This condition affects about a fourth of the older women in this country. It hits after menopause, when the body stops making its own estrogen. Estrogen, earlier in life, helps the body to make use of calcium for strong bones. If a woman has osteoporosis, her bones start losing calcium and get weak. This weakening leads to broken bones, a "hunchback," and other problems.

You know, sometimes you hear people say of an older

woman, "She slipped and broke her leg." But that's not true. What happened is this—her leg broke and *then* she slipped. That is often the way that women find out they have osteoporosis.

There is a lot of controversy about the proper medical treatment for this condition. It is important for women to talk over treatment with their doctors.

But there is no controversy about the fact that exercise helps strengthen bones. Exercise is a crucial part of treatment. It is essential! It allows the body to use the calcium to make bones strong. NASA once developed a machine called a *bone analyzer*. They wanted to find out how travel in space affected the astronauts' bones. They discovered that exercise is the best thing to make strong bones.

Since nobody can predict—male or female—whether or not they will get osteoporosis, it is a good idea to start exercising *at any age*. Exercise is the best prevention.

13

One Thing Leads to Another: My Video and Weight Control

Sharing Sensible Exercise

My exercise class was becoming really popular. I got carried away with the idea of more people hearing my story. My son suggested that we could make a videotape of the exercises and then people all over the country could fight back against arthritis.

"I don't have that kind of money," I said to him, trying to imagine buying an entire TV studio.

"Well, Dad, it only costs six hundred dollars to buy a video camera."

"I don't have a spare six hundred dollars anywhere," I said to him. "Who could help us?"

"The Thomsen agency advertises itself as a full-service agency. Maybe they do videos."

Mitchell is a small town. Everybody knows all the businesses. We went out to the advertising agency. And they agreed to help us spread the word. I guess most people think that seniors don't exercise. Maybe it's unusual to see all of us staying active.

So the Thomsen agency made a videotape and now it is being used by people all over the country, in senior centers, homes, apartment complexes, etc.

My Video and My Weight Control

What I enjoy about life is how you can't ever tell what's going to happen next. I wanted to make the videotape to spread the word about sensible, slow-moving exercise. But what happened after that was I saw myself on video and decided I needed to do something about my weight. I didn't expect to have that reaction!

They say that TV adds ten pounds to a person's weight. If you ever see my tape, I want you to remember that. I'm not as overweight as I look.

I've known for a long time I should do something about my weight. *Everybody* who has arthritis has heard along the way that it's a good idea to slim down. Because weight adds stress to the joints. I knew that but I wasn't motivated, even after years of exercise.

Weight adds stress to the joints. One of the best things you can do for yourself is take a load off your feet and sit down and rest during the day and get that extra weight off! That's why it's also true that swimming and riding an exercise bike are good exercise for people with arthritis. It's exercise without putting stress on our joints.

I started cutting down on my calories. No crazy fad diet. Just cutting down. That's hard work around my house. My wife Leona takes good care of me. Too good. She's a great German cook and I'm an Irishman, which means I'll eat anything! But it's possible for even an Irishman to cut back. I looked in the mirror and saw a man who weighed 206 pounds and I knew the time had come. My excess weight was causing a great deal of pain in my knees and ankles when I walked. My doctor at the VA told me I should start cutting back on my calories.

I guess I simply hadn't been ready to do the work before this time. I had spent many years working at my recovery—the exercising and getting myself to the whirlpool every day took all my concentration. I had not yet been ready to work at my eating habits. I believe that each of us is on a separate journey—we can only work on one change at a time. But now I was ready to tackle this next problem. Many other people will be able to get their weight down first and then exercise. I'm not saying that my way is the right way—it was just my way, the way I had to do it.

I had done enough reading to know I had to cut back on calories. At that time, I was eating six slices of bread a day. I decided to go to meetings of a class called Sensible Eating to get some moral support for my calorie-counting. That was a great help.

The class reinforced what I'd learned in my reading and at health fairs—that seniors should eat a *healthy* diet before thinking about weight loss. I had to make some changes with regard to my *health*, not just my weight. That's what the word *sensible* means.

Some people believe that diet can affect their arthritis. I don't myself believe this. But some people swear by it. Maybe it's true for them. The book *Natural Relief for Arthritis* (see page 67) goes into great detail about several diets. Apparently people with gout can get a great deal of relief by watching what they eat.

But the plan I followed is a plan for my general overall health and eventual weight loss. Seniors need to eat less, because our metabolism has slowed down and we don't burn calories as fast. This means that it is all the more important for us to eat nutritious food. We are the last people on earth who should be eating the "empty calories" of white sugar—pop, jelly rolls, alcohol! Here are some *DOS* and *DON'TS* I followed in order to be a healthier person:

DOS:
- Make sure you have good protein every day. Include fish, chicken, beans, rather than steaks.

- Include whole foods as much as possible—whole wheat bread, rather than white bread, homemade meals rather than TV dinners. Maybe friends can plan a potluck and each person will only have to fix one dish. That way a whole meal can come into being.

- Go shopping for fresh fruits and vegetables and *eat them*! (Don't let them rot in the refrigerator.)

- To help your digestion, which has also slowed down, drink more fluids than earlier in your life and eat foods with fiber. (These foods include whole-grain breads and cereals, raw fruits and vegetables.)

- *Drink more water!*

- Check to see that you have calcium in your diet *every day*. Your bones need it.

DON'TS:
- Don't add salt to your food. Cut back as much as possible. Read the labels in the grocery store and look for products that say LOW SODIUM.

- Don't eat white, refined sugar. Try eating an apple instead of that caramel roll!

- Don't eat much fat. Watch out for fried foods, foods with saturated fat, *all junk food*.

- If you take a vitamin and mineral supplement, *never* take more than a daily dose. You can read the label to see if the tablet is 100 percent RDA (Required Daily Allowance).

• Watch your alcohol! Don't overdo. Alcohol is empty calories and gives us nothing but a beer belly!

I followed these *Dos* and *Don'ts*. Of course, it took time to make these changes. But I look at it this way: Seniors have got the time! Of all the people alive in this country, seniors are the ones with time. We're fresh out of excuses for eating junk food! We can make one small change every day. Decide to cut up an apple for a snack instead of reaching for that bag of potato chips.

It takes a great deal of willpower and determination to refrain from eating. But I was determined, as usual. Once I started, I got out my old Harbert stubbornness. I made changes in my life. When I sent out to a restaurant, I no longer ordered anything that was deep-fat fried. I looked for something good that was broiled. I ordered a dinner salad instead of going to the salad bar and loading up on all that potato salad with mayonnaise! Then, after I had made some of these changes for my health, I started counting calories. I got a chart to keep track of what I had to eat every day. I dug out a small scale that weighed ounces. I bought lean steaks and cut them in three-ounce pieces. And then I limited myself to that much meat per day. I couldn't give up red meat totally!

I continued to read about food. I got a little book that lists the calorie content of every food from A to Z. I continued to go to my Sensible Eating group for support. Taking the time to go to a group is a big change in and of itself. And soon I started losing weight. It was a long struggle. But over the course of about two years, I went from 206 pounds to my present weight of 165.

I did myself a big favor in this struggle. I feel better now than ever. Sensible exercise and sensible eating are now a part of my life and life-style. I couldn't go back to sitting around and I couldn't go back to junk food! I feel too good!

If this chapter has inspired you to take a look at your eating habits, you need to go to your doctor for both a checkup and a talk about nutrition. Nobody should make changes in their diet and life-style without first talking to their doctor!

14

Fresh Out of Excuses: How Other People Have Used My Program

People have all kinds of excuses for not exercising. I thought maybe if I listed some of the excuses I've heard from people _before_ they started my program, you could see that you are not alone. If all the people in my classes made this big change, so can you.

I'm going to list some excuses I've heard—and my responses to them. Maybe you'll get a kick out of the way people think. We're all in the same boat. We have to work up the energy to make a change. We all use excuses all the time.

I don't have time.
You may not have the time now, but you can _make_ time. You can make the time by _taking the time_. Just give up one sedentary activity.

What's the point? I'm already out of shape!
For one thing, you'll look better. Most people would like to look better. I know one woman who refused to exercise until a younger man caught her eye!

It's too late.
This one's easy. I bet you already know what I'll say: *it's never too late!*

It hurts.
True enough. It may hurt. But if you keep living a sedentary life, the hurting is going to get worse. There are many ways to deal with pain and you can find a way that works for you to diminish pain. You can find a way to relax before you start exercising and then it won't hurt as much. Take care of yourself and the pain will diminish.

I have a full schedule already.
This excuse is a variation on *I don't have time.* Maybe a person who uses the word *schedule* simply needs to write the word *exercise* into their schedule! Then it will be part of the full schedule.

I have too many other people to take care of.
You are the most important person for you to take care of. If *your* body falls apart, how will you be of any use whatsoever to anyone else?

I don't know anybody else who exercises.
Maybe it's time for you to meet some new friends! If you go to an exercise class, you will then know some people who exercise.

I have no reason to exercise.
There has to be *something* that you would like to do that *you* can think of as reason to motivate yourself: something as simple as walking in the woods for mushrooms in the fall—or something as strenuous as gardening again.

I can't do it.
If a totally disabled man can fight his way back to mobility and mental health, so can you!

I've heard all these excuses many times. And I've seen people forget them, easily, once they start exercising. They're fresh out of excuses and they love it!

I'd like to tell you about some of the people who have used my program and how it's become a part of their lives.

You remember the story of my friend Anna Uhrich? She picked me up on the road to recovery and introduced me to square dancing. I also went to the exercise classes at the Y with Anna. When I took over the class several years later, she kept coming. So I have had a chance to repay her some of the kindness she showed me. She has terrible arthritis, and she still comes to my class when she is in town. She often goes visiting her grown-up children. Her exercising keeps her on the go—her hands are swollen with arthritis but she doesn't let it slow her down. If you ever get a chance to see my tape *Sensible Exercise*, you will see her. The camera shows a close-up of her hands. Anna leads an active, happy life.

Another woman in Mitchell who started coming to my class was so crippled up that she could not even bend over to pick up a quart of milk on her back stoop. She had terrible arthritis and back trouble. She had to start out exercising *very slowly* and *very gradually*. She was in a lot of pain. She could hardly lift her arms. She couldn't bend over at all. Gradually, her muscles grew stronger and her joints became more flexible. Now she is able to move freely, walk where she wants to go. Now she can do her favorite thing again—gardening. She weeds, hoes, harvests, picks her beans! She has such a plentiful garden that she brings vegetables to our class as gifts to all of us.

She changed from a disabled person to an active person within the short period of two years.

I've seen other amazing success stories. But I want to point out, again, that not all the successes are physical. We also have success with our mental attitude when we are exercising. After my class, everyone feels so happy that we go to the cafeteria and have a cup of coffee and visit. Yes, we have *decaf*. We have to watch our caffeine intake. Exercising and socializing seem to go hand in hand. I've noticed that people look happy as we're finishing the class with the exercise of giving a neck rub to the person in front of us. Since most seniors live alone, it has occurred to me that the exercise class might be the only time during the day that some of us are able to touch or hug another person. That friendly physical contact has a lot to do with our well-being. As I mentioned before, loneliness and depression are issues of concern to many seniors.

My friends on the staff of the Mitchell Senior Center say that one of the good things about my exercise program is the fact that people stay and visit. I'm better than bingo!

The videotape that we made of my program is being sold now to individuals and to centers and to other places where seniors gather. It is my hope that people will use my book to exercise at home and then find a place where they can get out and exercise with other people.

We are just beginning to hear from people about how they are using my program. The senior centers are generally using the tape for exercise classes *and* letting the tape be checked out by people who want to use it at home. Some of the staff of the senior centers are taking the tape around to health fairs to try to raise peoples' awareness of the need for exercise for seniors.

One woman recently wrote to us about how much her class liked my tape. She said it was their favorite of the many on the market. Her class dubbed my tape "The Old Man." She said they liked it the best because it was more their style and speed—they are in their seventies and eighties. And that's exactly what I've discovered with my own classes. I'm not a Superman bodybuilder—just an ordinary senior citizen who wants to do the best I can with what I've got!

Another woman wrote that she played the tape at her senior center where people were waiting to be served their noon meal. She wanted to see if there was any interest in a class. The seniors responded very positively— they got up from the table and started exercising along with me! How's that for spontaneous enthusiasm! This woman recommends that all senior centers serving meals at noon also offer an exercise class.

Of course, the problem for the centers is funding. Many centers barely have funds to cover the programs that are already going. So this becomes a problem for the larger community. A political problem. What is happening to our seniors? Does anybody out there care?

One woman who cares is Pam Schelir, of Madera, California. She is an assemblywoman of Fresno and Madera County. She is an activist for the rights and concerns of seniors. She believes that the larger community should provide the opportunity for seniors to exercise—at their centers, housing complexes, etc. If only funding were available or the tapes donated, the idea of exercise might catch on and spread like wildfire. Pam says that exercise is crucial for physical and mental health. Pam points out that even though the brain is only 2 percent of our body volume, it uses 20 percent of the oxygen we take in. Oxygen keeps us mentally alive! New research shows that exercise will improve the existing mental functions of people with Alzheimer's disease. I'm not surprised by this new research. It backs up what I've noticed all along— *everybody* does better if they exercise. No matter what diseases or conditions we have, we will do better all the way around if we exercise.

It looks like my tape is getting people to think more about exercise and seniors. I guess nobody ever saw an exercise tape before that had such ordinary people in it as my friends and neighbors from Mitchell, South Dakota. CBS news came out and covered my class and the broadcaster said, "Virgil's exercise video isn't slick, but, then, neither is Virgil." How true! You don't have to be slick to be healthy! I'm an ordinary person and my aim is to reach out and help all the other ordinary people who are suffering from arthritis and other disabilities. More power to us!

15

Be Patient: God Isn't Through with Me Yet: My Life Today

Change Is a Sign of Life

Whenever I think of that sign in the Senior Center, BE PATIENT: GOD ISN'T THROUGH WITH ME YET, I have to chuckle, because I keep going through changes. I could never have imagined the changes I've been through. When I was sixty-one, I thought my life was over, I never imagined I could recover as well as I have. When I was sixty-seven, I was in better shape, but I never imagined myself as the Exercise Guru! Now at age seventy-one, I'm seeing myself look forward to more changes. I love to hear stories about older people who take up something for the first time. Did you know that Laura Ingalls Wilder started her "Little House" books when she was around seventy years old? Think of what she gave us. Think about all the people whose lives have been happier

97

because of her books. Think about all those kids watching TV re-runs. She didn't sit down in her rocking chair and wait around to die. God wasn't through with her yet.

My Life This Year

Leona and I live in a little house in Mitchell, on First Avenue, the very street where my parents lived when I was born. "Our shack," I call it, because it's so little. But, then, both of us are short. I'm even smaller since I got my weight under control.

You may wonder how my arthritis is now. Well, I never promised myself a cure. My arthritis is still with me. It is my companion, but I don't let it run my life. It wakes me up in the night, no doubt about it. Sometimes I have to get up two times in a night. I rub lineament on my knees and walk around a bit. I've had to cut back on some activities. Dancing. How I love dancing! But my knees can't take it anymore. The backs of my knees hurt when I go dancing, unless I have a drink or two, and I don't want to get in that habit. So we only go dancing a couple of times a year.

But my arthritis doesn't slow me down much. I get up in the morning ready to go. I go to the Y everyday and sit in the whirlpool and do my own exercises. Then I teach my class three mornings a week at the Senior Center. Then I teach in the afternoon, three times a week, at the Brady Memorial Home. In between my classes, I go to my part-time job as an aide at the school for the kids getting on and off the school buses. Sitting around isn't good for me. I have to do something. Besides, I've got bills to pay. Leona just had open-heart surgery and you wouldn't believe the bills. Well, maybe you would believe them. Still, we have our health and we're happy.

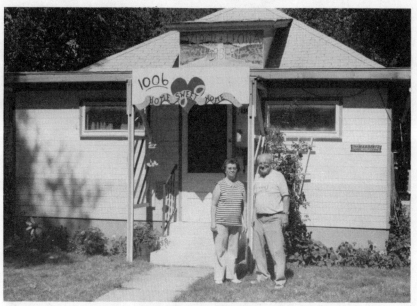

*This is our shack—I painted
the signs myself.*

Working with People
in Wheelchairs

The biggest change in my life recently is my class for people in wheelchairs at the Brady Memorial Home.

I go out there three times a week and we have fun! People in wheelchairs are the same as people out of chairs—they like to have company, and they need to exercise. And most of all, they like to laugh! They like my jokes. I don't understand prejudice against disabled people. Anybody can have their body go out on them. It can happen to anyone. That doesn't change your basic human needs and your sense of humor.

So I've adapted the exercises to work for people sitting down. I've added some new ones, to have something different to do when I go out there. When I lead the class, I encourage *everyone* to try—some of the older people who get wheeled in look feeble, but after a while, they get into the swing of it. I say, "If you can't lift your arms, at least count along with me." Some people have turned in

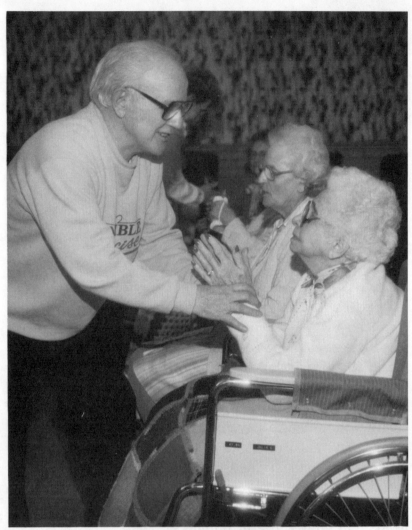

Even people in wheelchairs need exercise—and they enjoy it in my class!

so on themselves that even talking is a big effort. Our voices are part of our bodies. Using our voices can be a first step to using our bodies more.

Some people take part by sitting and watching and counting out loud with me. Others can count and wave their hands—they can't bend or lift their arms, but they're doing something good for themselves.

When I watch the slow improvement of some, I see again that slow, small movements are important and worthwhile. One woman started doing finger exercises and gradually moved on to arm exercises. She got better and stronger. More than that, she has some hope. She didn't give up and sit in her chair, depressed.

I like to tell my jokes out there, just as much as anywhere. I try to make the directions for the exercises funny, like saying, "Let's shovel snow out of the driveway," rather than "Let's swing our arms." One day I came out to class, wearing a pig nose. I spent most of my life with animals, so I must say that I can do a pretty good imitation of most animal sounds. When I act silly, people loosen up and giggle and relax about their attempts to exercise.

There are some people there who have Alzheimer's disease. I'm not sure if they are aware of us. But, maybe they can sense our company and know that we care about them. I feel a sense of community with the people at the home.

It's good for me to get out and volunteer. It gets my energy going. Change is a sign of life. I think every older person ought to consider doing some kind of volunteer work.

Of Service to Others

Right now, teaching the exercises classes is my main volunteer work. But over the years, I've done quite a few

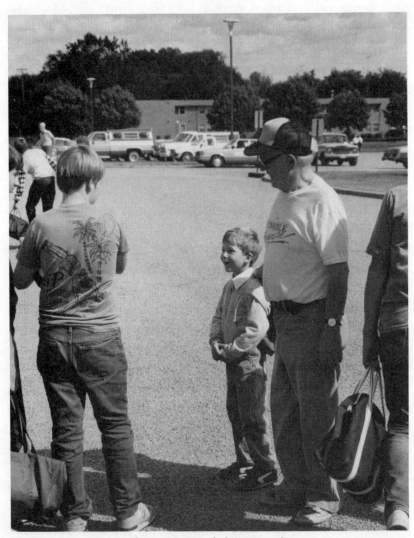

I like to get out and about every day.

other things. I've had fun! No matter whether we're disabled or able-bodied, it's good for us to get out and see
people. What better way to see people than to help out
somewhere. There always something that needs doing.
When we're seniors, we may not have much money, but
we usually have some free time. Remember: Change is a
sign of life. When you try something new, it's a sign that
there's still some life left in you.

I've done lots of volunteer work. I've worked with
kids. I often play Santa Claus for preschoolers. One year
I developed a Santa Claus clown act. At Halloween, the
Modern Woodmen put on a party at the Corn Palace to
keep the kids off the street. I helped with that for four
years. Sometimes I help baby-sit when the Christian
Women's Club has a luncheon. And so forth.

And then there's the Senior Center. I've been a
handyman around the place. I mowed the lawn for three
years. I served on the Board. I also did Meals on Wheels
for three years; that is, I did the driving to deliver the
meals, I didn't do the cooking. Sometimes I helped with
other kinds of errands.

I've even gotten awards for my volunteer work. But
there are plenty of others in our town who deserve
awards and who have never been recognized. We have
over three hundred volunteers in our seniors' organization. So I'm not claiming to be unique—I am only one of
the many—an ordinary guy doing my bit to help make life
more pleasant. I've got energy to burn. Why not be
useful?

I also like to think that when I get old, someone will
be there for me.

What could you do in your community? We may be
disabled, we may be retired, but we're not dead yet! God
isn't done with us yet.

103

Still Dreaming Today

All scientific research all over our country has said that exercise is worthwhile, especially for older people. But too many seniors are sitting and playing cards or bingo until the day that I am hauling Meals on Wheels to them. And I'm the one who was totally disabled!

I wish I could see more of my friends leading active lives. I've had to learn the hard way. As I mentioned before, I joke about reading George Burns's book, *How to Live to Be 100 or Older*. He says he surrounds himself with beautiful women. That's what I'm doing! Like I said, most of the people who come to my class are women and I love them all. It makes no difference if they're short, fat, tall, or skinny. I think they're all beautiful. They are loving, caring people who raised their families. They have paid their dues, too. They deserve to stay happy and healthy on God's good green earth for many years. I am trying to help them and help myself at the same time.

I think about all those years I was sitting out on the farm, dreaming about making a success of my life as a farmer. I'm still dreaming—only now I'm dreaming of older Americans learning how to exercise and have a happy life. I'm dreaming of many of us winning the fight against arthritis. I'm still dreaming. It's never too late.

Exercise Section

Getting Ready to Exercise

Before you start any exercise program, you should see the doctor for a checkup. Ask the doctor if it is OK for you to exercise.

Many people already have an individual exercise program, designed by a physical therapist or a doctor. These people should also ask about adding any of my exercises to their routine.

Respect your body! See the doctor!

Here are the things to remember when you start my exercise program:

1. Wear loose, warm clothing. Wear *comfortable* clothes.

2. Wear shoes *and socks*. Nylon stockings don't count as socks! Make sure the soles of your shoes are a nonslip material.

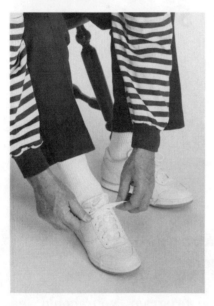 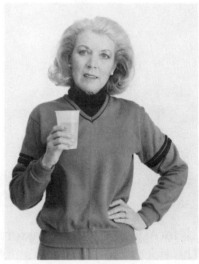

3. Remember to drink some water *before* and after exercising. It really is important to increase your water intake.

4. Stand up straight, keep your back straight.

   Don't arch your back or twist your body into awkward positions—don't get bent out of shape!

   Keep your knees slightly bent—not rigid.

5. Move SLOWLY and DELIBERATELY! DON'T BOUNCE. Small, gentle motions work!

6. If you are a beginner, don't try to do the entire exercise routine all at once.

Do each exercise two or three times and then rest. Frozen joints need to be worked slowly to loosen up. Don't push it!

7. If you are having a flare-up of your arthritis, take it easy. You may want to do each exercise once, in order to keep your present range of motion. Then let yourself rest for a few days.

8. Be sure you breathe normally while exercising. DON'T EVER HOLD YOUR BREATH! It's OK to stop and breathe if you think you're out of breath. See exercise 3 (which follows).

   It is important to take in lots of air when we exercise!

So now we should be ready to begin. If you have followed all my instructions, you are ready to go.
   But first, a few last-minute cautions:

• If you have muscle cramping during any exercise, it's OK to STOP! Rub the cramped muscle. Continue with slower, easier movements.

• If you start to feel sick, STOP. (By *sick* I mean: *dizzy, woozy, chest pain, sick to your stomach*.)

• If you are having more pain in your joints than is usual, STOP.

• If you need to breathe, STOP AND BREATHE. Rest before you continue.

Let's start out with some simple warmups. Remember, if a disabled man can do these, you can, too. Be patient with yourself. If you are stiff, your muscles weak, just try each exercise one time through in the beginning.

1 | *Reach and Stretch*

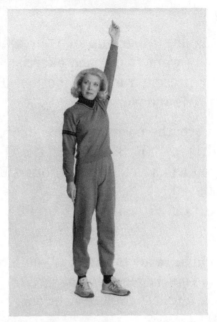

1. Reach up high with your left arm. Reach for the ceiling.

2. Keep your arm straight as you reach up.

3. Lower your arm in front of you, keeping the elbow straight as your arm comes down. Then let it rest at your side.

Count 1 as your arm is going up.

Count 2 as your arm is coming down.

Count to 20, doing the exercise completely 10 times.

Repeat the exercise with your right arm, following the directions.

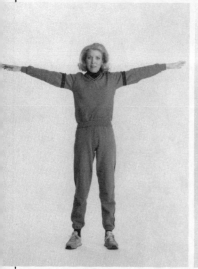 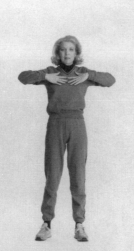 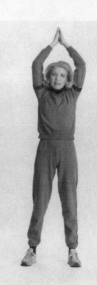

1. Hold your arms out to your sides at shoulder level.

2. Bend your arms at the elbow and bring the palms of your hands to your chest.

3. Extend your arms out straight again.

4. Raise your arms high over your head and touch your hands together.

5. Repeat the exercise.

Count 1 as you extend your arms.

Count 2 as you move your hands to your chest.

Count 3 as you extend your arms again.

Count 4 as you raise your arms over your head.

Count 5 as you extend your arms, and so on.

Count until you reach 40.

3 | *Deep Breathing*

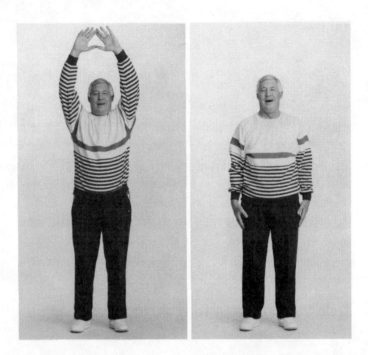

1. Breathe in and raise your arms up from your sides until your hands are high over your head.

2. Exhale through your mouth as you slowly let your arms come down. Rest your arms at your sides.

Count 1 as your arms go up.

Count 2 as your arms come down.

Keep counting, 3, up—4, down—until you have reached 10.

Bubble Gum Chewing | 4

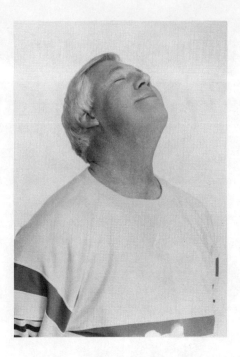

1. Tip your head back, far enough so you can see the ceiling.

2. Pretend to be chewing bubble gum—or chewing tobacco!

Count up to 20. Chomp, jaw, chew!

You won't be able to count out loud.

5 *Massage Your Neck*

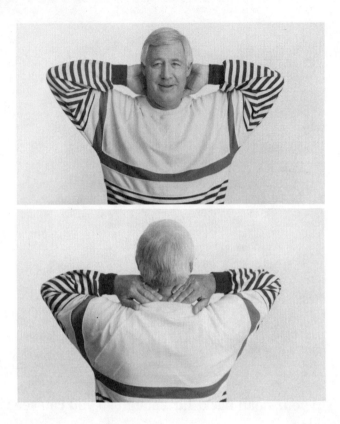

1. Lift your hands to your neck. Put your fingers on the back of your neck.

2. Rub your neck muscles slowly and gently and strongly.

Rub your neck for 1 minute.

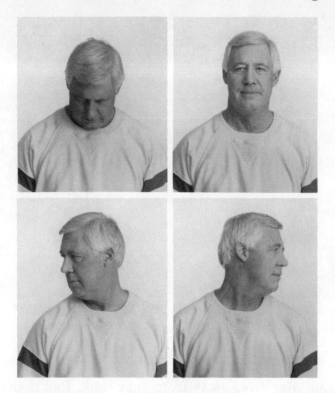

1. Drop your chin to your chest. Look at the floor. Then raise it again, so you're looking straight ahead.

2. Turn your head slowly to the right as far as you can. Keep your head up as you turn. Don't look down.

3. Look forward again.

4. Turn your head slowly to the left as far as you can. Go gently. Don't strain your muscles. Stop when you have reached your limit.

Go through all these motions 4 times.

7 | Hands Behind Back: Guess Which Hand It's In

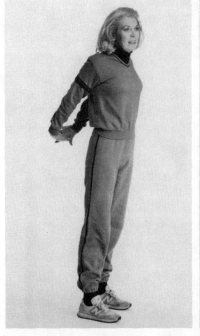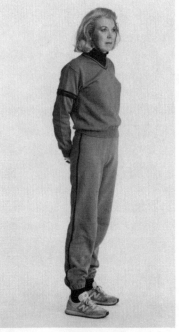

1. Clasp your hands behind you.

2. Lift your arms away from your back. Pull back gently. You may bend forward slightly.

3. Relax your arms and lower your clasped hands.

Count 1 as you lift your arms.

Count 2 as you let your arms fall back.

Count until you reach 20.

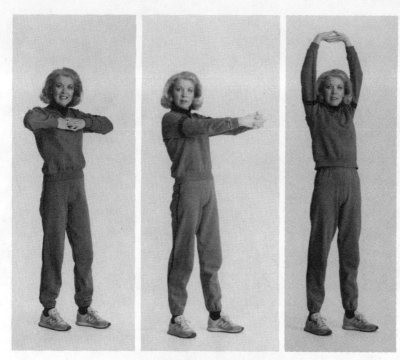

1. Lace your fingers together on your chest (Keep them laced throughout the exercise). Push your arms straight out in front of you.

2. Bring your arms back to your chest.

3. Turn your hands so your palms are facing out. Reach towards the ceiling with your palms out, still keeping your fingers laced.

4. Bring your arms back to the original position on your chest.

Count with the numbers as they are listed above.

When you start over, count 5, 6, 7, 8.

Count to 20. Then you will have done the exercise 5 times.

9 | *Arms Wrapped Overhead*

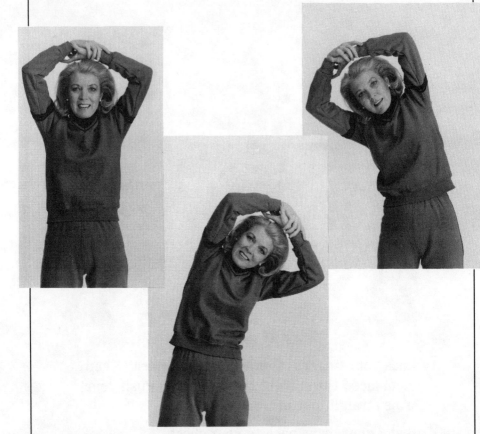

1. Put your arms on top of your head, with your hands grasping your wrists, forearms, or elbows.

2. Hold your arms still and bend gently to one side from the waist.

3. Then bend to the other side.

Count very slowly.

Count 1 as you bend to one side.

Count 2 as you bend to the other side.

Count to 10.

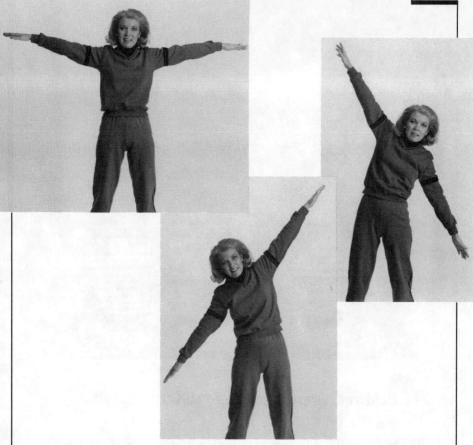

1. Extend your arms out to your sides at shoulder level and bend slowly to one side from your waist. Count slowly from 1 to 10. 1, 2, 3, 4, 5, 6, 7, 8, 9, 10.

2. While you are bending, keep your arms straight like a teeter-totter.

3. Then bend to the other side and count to 10.

Do this exercise 3 times.

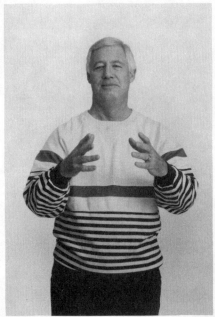 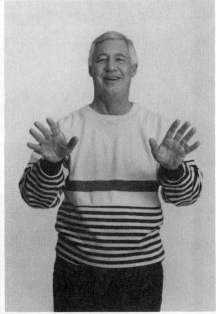

1. Hold your arms in front of you with your elbows slightly bent.

2. Make circular motions with your hands. Just let your hands relax and move with your wrists.

3. Now make circles in the other direction.

Do 20 circles each way.

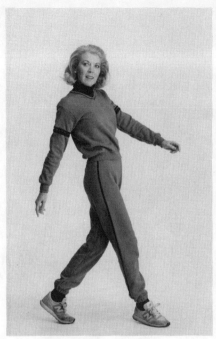 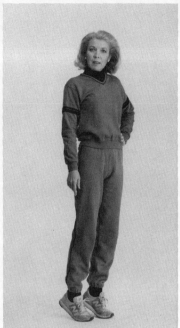

1. Stand with your feet together and then step as far forward with your right foot as is comfortable.

2. Bring your right foot back, so that you're standing with your feet together again.

3. Now stand on your tip-toes—both feet.

4. Lower yourself down so you're standing flat on the ground again. You are now back at the starting position.

5. Now step forward with your left foot . . .

Count 1, 2, 3, 4, along with the directions above.

When you start with your left foot, say 5, and so forth, until you reach 40.

13 *Shoulder Rolls*

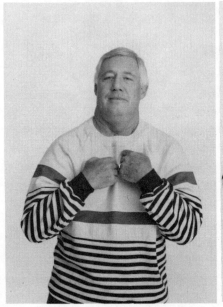 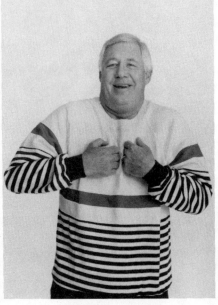

1. Place your hands on your chest, fingers closed. Keep your arms relaxed, elbows at your sides.

2. Roll your shoulders forward in a circular motion— forward, up, around, down, and forward again.

Make 10 circles forward and then 10 circles backward.

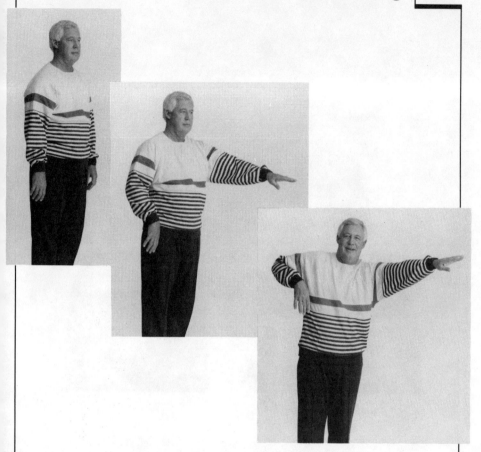

1. Start with your hands at your sides. Bending your elbow, slide one arm up your side as far as you can and then stretch the arm out in front of you, as if you were swimming. Reach as far as you can and then lower your arm to your side.

2. While one arm is sliding up your side, the other arm will be reaching out. Pretend you're doing the Australian crawl.

Count 1 as you slide your arm up your side, 2 as you stretch and lower it, and so forth. Count to 20.

15 *Shoulders to Ears*

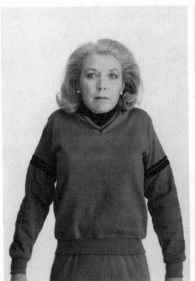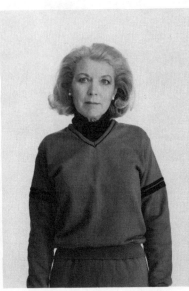

1. Hunch your shoulders up to your ears slowly.

2. Hold your shoulders in the up position.

3. Slowly let your shoulders relax and return to their normal position.

Count 1 as your shoulders go up.

Count 2 as you hold them up.

Count 3 as they come down.

Count to 30.

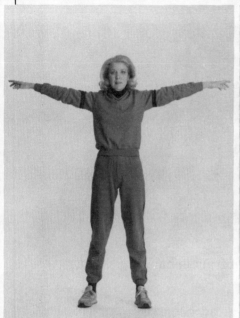 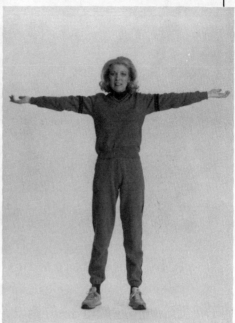

1. Extend your arms straight out to the sides at shoulder level, palms down.

2. Keep your arms in the same position, and turn your palms up.

Count 1 for palms down.

Count 2 for palms up.

Count 3 for palms down.

Count 4 for palms up.

Count to 20.

17 | *Wiggle and Close: Finger Exercises*

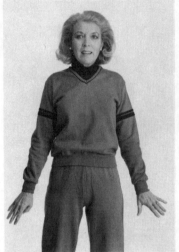 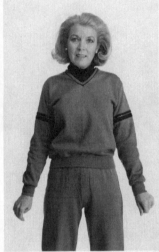 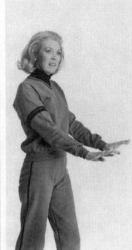

1. Do this exercise with your arms hanging at your sides.

2. Wiggle your fingers for a few seconds.

3. Now make fists with both hands.

4. Repeat 4 more times.

5. Now shake 'em out. Shake your hands in a relaxed way, as though you were shaking water off.

6. Now hold your arms in front of you, at waist level, and repeat the exercise.

Instead of counting, we say, "Wiggle . . . close . . ." in a regular rhythm.

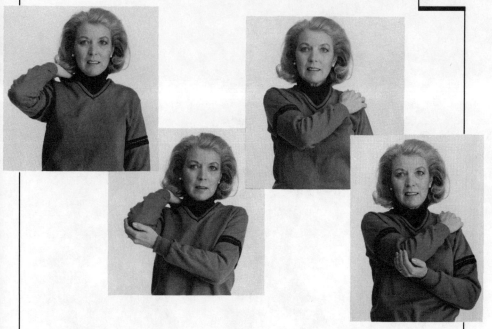

1. Bend your right arm and touch your right shoulder.

2. Use your left hand to give support to your right arm by holding your elbow and lifting a little.

3. Let your arms fall to your side.

4. Reach your right arm across your chest and pat your left shoulder—hold your elbow again.

5. Go back to the beginning and pat yourself on the right shoulder.

Count 1 for the touching and lifting.

Count 2 for letting your arms fall down.

Count 3 for touching and lifting the other shoulder.

Count from 1 to 20.

Repeat with the other arm.

19 | *Knee Bends*

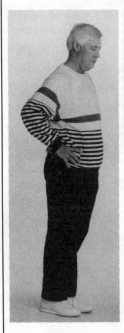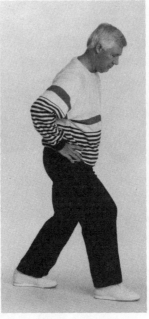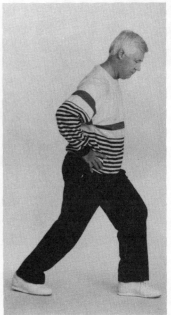

1. Stand in a relaxed position, with your hands on your waist.

2. Step forward with your right foot and bend your knee a little bit. Keep the heel of your left foot on the ground!

3. Bring your foot back to the starting position.

4. Do this 5 times.

Count 1 for stepping forward.

Count 2 for coming back.

Count to 10.

Repeat with the other foot.

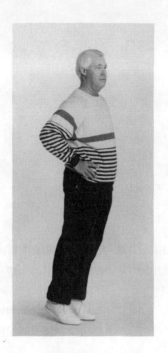

1. Stand in a relaxed position with your feet together.

2. Rise slowly up on your tip-toes.

3. Then lower yourself slowly until you're standing with your heels on the ground again.

Count 1 for up.

Count 2 for down.

Count to 20.

21 | *Walking for 1 Minute*

This is an easy one! Just walk around the room for 1 minute—be sure to time it because it may seem like a long time. This walking gives your body a chance to slow down, cool down, and relax. At the end of the minute, find a sturdy kitchen chair for the following exercises.

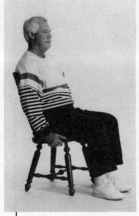 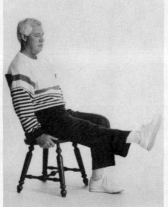 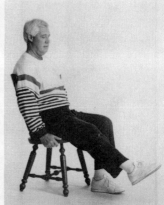

1. Sit up straight in the chair facing forward, with your feet flat on the floor.

2. Lift your right leg up a few inches off the floor.

3. Now straighten your leg as much as you can and stretch.

4. Bend your leg again and keep your foot off the floor.

5. Lower your leg to the floor.

6. Do this 5 times.

Count 1 for lifting your leg up.

Count 2 for stretching it out.

Count 3 for bending your knee.

Count 4 for lowering your leg.

Count 5 for starting over.

Count 1 to 20.

Repeat with the left leg.

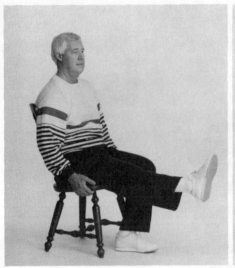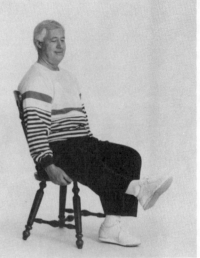

1. Sit up straight in the chair, feet flat on the floor.

2. Lift your right leg off the floor and stretch it straight out in front of you.

3. Move it as far to your right as you can.

4. Now move it back so that it's straight out in front of you, still up in the air, at the level of the chair.

Count 1 for waving sideways.

Count 2 for coming back.

Count 1 to 10.

---

1. Now point your toe and do the same exercise as listed above: this is called WAVING THE LEG WITH THE TOE POINTED. It exercises different muscles.

Repeat this exercise with the left leg.

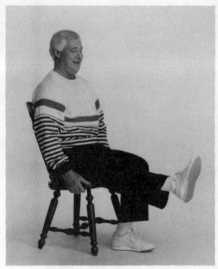 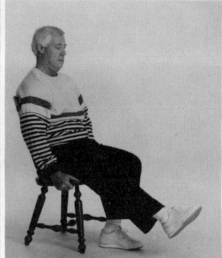

1. Sit in the chair. Relax. Sit up straight!

2. Lift your right leg off the floor and stretch it out in front of you.

3. Make small circles with your leg.

4. Make 5 circles one way and then reverse the direction and make 5 circles the other way.

Repeat this exercise with the left leg.

25 | *Elbows on Knees*

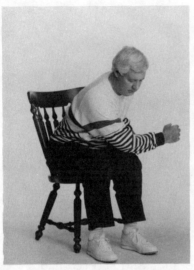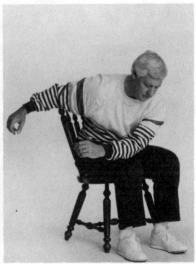

1. Sit straight up in the chair and relax.

2. Hold your hands in front of your chest and lift your bent elbows until they're at shoulder level.

3. Lean over now and try to touch your left knee with your right elbow.

4. Straighten up and then lean over and try to touch your right knee with your left elbow.

Count 1 for the first touch.

Count 2 for the second touch, etc. Stretch gently— don't strain!

Count from 1 to 20.

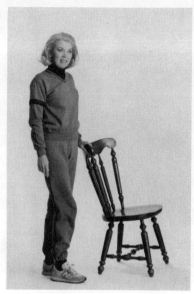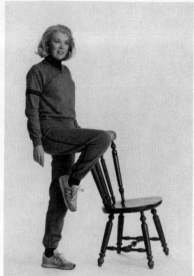

1. Stand beside the chair. Turn it so you can use the back to support you.

2. Hold on to the back of the chair with your left hand.

3. Lift your right leg up and bend your knee. You will look like you're getting ready to pedal a bike.

4. Lower your leg and stand still for a moment.

Count 1 as you lift your leg.

Count 2 as you lower it.

Count 3 as you lift it again.

Count from 1 to 20.

Repeat this exercise with your left leg.

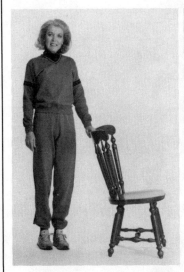 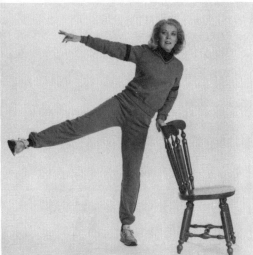

1. Turn your chair so you can hold on to the back with your left hand for support.

2. Lift your right leg out from your side and up. (This is not a forward kick.)

3. As you lift, raise your right arm in the air also, as high as you can.

4. Move your leg very slowly. It's OK *if you only move it a few inches*.

Count 1 for going up.

Count 2 for coming down.

Count from 1 to 20.

Repeat this exercise with the left leg.

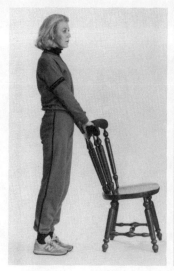 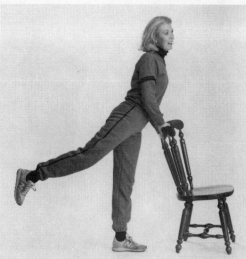

1. Stand facing the back of the chair and hold onto it with both hands.

2. Slowly kick backward—first one leg and then the other.

Count 1 for the right leg going up.

Count 2 for it coming down.

Count 3 for the left leg going up.

Count 4 for it coming down, etc.

Count from 1 to 20.

Reaching Toward the Knees

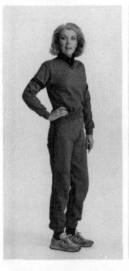 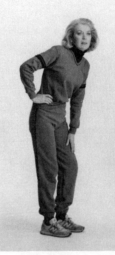 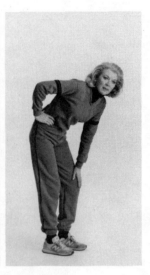

1. Stand in a relaxed position, with your knees slightly bent.

2. Bend sideways and slide your left hand down your left leg, toward your knee—if you reach it, fine, if not, just reach in that direction. Stretch but don't strain yourself.

3. Return to the standing position.

4. Bend over and reach again.

Count 1 for reaching toward the right knee.

Count 2 when you straighten up.

Count 3 when you reach down again.

Count from 1 to 10.

Repeat the exercise sliding your right hand down your right leg, counting 1 to 10.

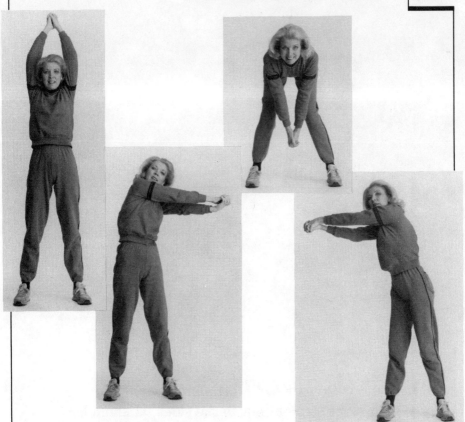

1. Hold your arms up over your head and clasp your hands together. Pretend your arms are the hands of a clock at noon or part of a windmill!

2. Now move your arms together (keep the hands clasped!) around the face of the clock until they're at noon again. (You can bend over when your hands are at six o'clock.)

Count 1 slowly, for the first circle you make.

Count 2 for the second, etc., up to 5, then reverse directions and make 5 circles going the other way.

31 *Waist Twist # 1*

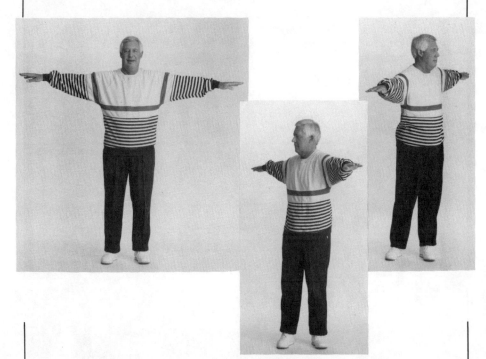

1. Stand with your feet a little bit apart. Extend your arms straight out to the sides, at shoulder level.

2. Keeping your arms straight throughout the exercise, turn from the waist to your right.

3. Face front again still keeping your arms out.

4. Turn from the waist to your left.

5. Now repeat . . .

Count 1 as you turn to the right.

Count 2 as you turn to the left, and so on.

Count slowly.

Count from 1 to 10.

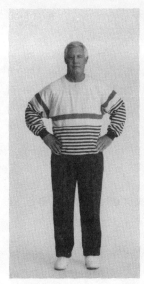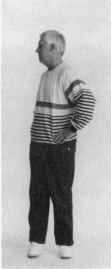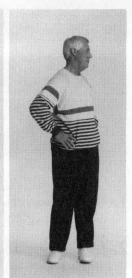

1. Place your hands on your hips and keep them there for the whole exercise. Feet flat on the floor!

2. Turn from the waist to the right as far as you can without straining.

3. Face front again and then turn left. Keep the motion smooth. Don't jerk!

Count 1 as you turn to the right.

Count 2 as you turn to the left.

Count slowly.

Count from 1 to 10.

33 | *Walk the Straight Line*

1. In this exercise, we let our bodies cool down by walking. Walk along an imaginary straight line.

2. If you run into an obstacle or a wall, make a right angle turn and walk the straight line in that direction.

3. Walk for about 1 minute to let your body relax.

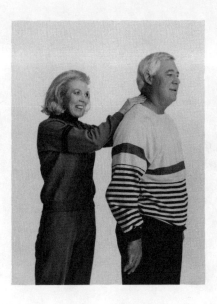

This is an exercise that you need a partner for!

1. After you've walked the straight line for a minute, walk close to another person. If there is a group exercising together, make a circle, so that each person can touch the person in front of him or her.

2. Walk in a circle slowly and massage gently the neck and shoulders of the person in front of you. If you are exercising with only one other person, you can take turns giving each other neck rubs.

35 *Step and Slide*

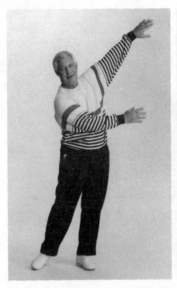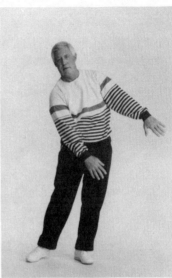

1. Step to the left with your left foot and swing your arms to the left as you step. Your weight is on your left foot, with your right heel slightly raised.

2. Then slide your right leg up next to your left leg.

3. Let your arms swing back to your sides as you slide.

Instead of counting, say out loud, "Step and slide."

Step, swing, and slide 10 times to your right, then do it 10 more times to your left.

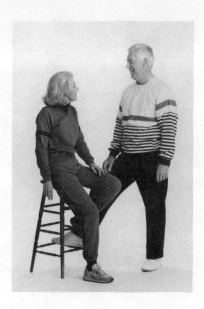

1. Sit down and rest for 5 minutes before starting any other activity.

2. Give yourself more resting time if you are on your way outdoors.

Now don't go away yet! Visit with your neighbor. Sit down and have some coffee. *Then* go out and have a good day! You deserve a healthy body and a happy life!